AIIMS May 2019
The Precise Version

AF515545

Celebrating 50 Years
Passion, Quality and Innovation in Healthcare Publishing

AIIMS May 2019
The Precise Version

Apurv Mehra
Leading Faculty of Orthopedics

Thameem Saif
Leading Faculty of Medicine

Akhil Monga
MD Radiodiagnosis, AIIMS

Vishnu Prasad
MD Radiodiagnosis, AIIMS

Chief Editors

Saurabh Taneja Consultant Critical Care at Sir Ganga Ram Hospital, New Delhi
Dipin Sudhakaran MD Radiodiagnosis, AIIMS, New Delhi
Amit Gupta MD Radiodiagnosis, AIIMS, New Delhi
Himanshu Gupta MD Radiodiagnosis, MAMC, New Delhi

JAYPEE

JAYPEE BROTHERS MEDICAL PUBLISHERS
The Health Sciences Publisher
New Delhi | London

Jaypee Brothers Medical Publishers (P) Ltd

Headquarters

Jaypee Brothers Medical Publishers (P) Ltd
4838/24, Ansari Road, Daryaganj
New Delhi 110 002, India
Phone: +91-11-43574357
Fax: +91-11-43574314
Email: jaypee@jaypeebrothers.com

Overseas Office

J.P. Medical Ltd
83 Victoria Street, London
SW1H 0HW (UK)
Phone: +44 20 3170 8910
Fax: +44 (0)20 3008 6180
Email: info@jpmedpub.com

Website: www.jaypeebrothers.com
Website: www.jaypeedigital.com

© 2019, Jaypee Brothers Medical Publishers

The views and opinions expressed in this book are solely those of the original contributor(s)/author(s) and do not necessarily represent those of editor(s) of the book.

All rights reserved. No part of this publication may be reproduced, stored or transmitted in any form or by any means, electronic, mechanical, photocopying, recording or otherwise, without the prior permission in writing of the publishers.

All brand names and product names used in this book are trade names, service marks, trademarks or registered trademarks of their respective owners. The publisher is not associated with any product or vendor mentioned in this book.

Medical knowledge and practice change constantly. This book is designed to provide accurate, authoritative information about the subject matter in question. However, readers are advised to check the most current information available on procedures included and check information from the manufacturer of each product to be administered, to verify the recommended dose, formula, method and duration of administration, adverse effects and contraindications. It is the responsibility of the practitioner to take all appropriate safety precautions. Neither the publisher nor the author(s)/editor(s) assume any liability for any injury and/ or damage to persons or property arising from or related to use of material in this book.

This book is sold on the understanding that the publisher is not engaged in providing professional medical services. If such advice or services are required, the services of a competent medical professional should be sought.

Every effort has been made where necessary to contact holders of copyright to obtain permission to reproduce copyright material. If any have been inadvertently overlooked, the publisher will be pleased to make the necessary arrangements at the first opportunity. The **CD/DVD-ROM** (if any) provided in the sealed envelope with this book is complimentary and free of cost. **Not meant for sale**.

Inquiries for bulk sales may be solicited at: jaypee@jaypeebrothers.com

AIIMS May 2019: The Precise Version

First Edition: **2019**

ISBN 978-93-89587-54-8

Printed at: Samrat Offset Pvt. Ltd.

MedMiracle
.... Empowers To Excel

Dedication

I dedicate this book to my students, my teachers and my patients who helped me evolve into a better teacher and Orthopedic Surgeon.

Apurv Mehra

I dedicate this book to all my students who have enabled me to become a better student of this awesome subject of medicine.

Thameem Saif

I dedicate this book to my parents.

Akhil Monga

I dedicate this book to my parents and Dr Aswani.

Vishnu Prasad

Teri Kismat da likha
Tere toh koi kho nahin sakda
Tu shram (Karam) kara chal bande…
Je usdi meher hove ta tenu o v mil jauga jo tera ho nahin sakda

Preface

Entrance exams are often seen as tough obstacles which are difficult to overcome. Exams can be easily taken care of once you identify the areas from which questions are asked. Assimilate the fact that you cannot study the whole syllabus of MBBS no matter how hard you try. Half the job is done once you pinpoint the hot topics to be focused upon. I would like to recommend a few tips to stay on the right track during your preparation:

- Avoid studying standard textbooks during your preparation, although you may use them for clearing your doubts—the reason being that they are difficult to revise.
- Choose one good review book per subject and use the same for revision—review books have the advantage of having only the most relevant topics.
- Special focus has to be given for 1st and 2nd year subjects, as they are mostly fact-based and high yielding.
- Subscribe to any one online test series which includes grand tests and subject wise tests and practice them regularly.
- Practice at least 20–30 questions daily.

Revision is the key to obtain a good rank. Once you attempt mock tests, you will realize that most of your answers come from your recent memory rather than your remote memory. Unless you revise things in the end, you will not be able to score well.

So, in this book we have compiled all the questions which have been in the May 2019 AIIMS entrance exam. All 200 questions have been included based on the most accurate recall. Correct answers and explanations have been taken from the standard textbooks. It is important to have a thorough reading of the whole book, as it will give you an idea about the hot topics that are frequently asked in AIIMS exams.

Wishing you good luck for your forthcoming exams!!

Apurv Mehra
Thameem Saif
Akhil Monga
Vishnu Prasad

Practice High Yield Authentic AIIMS Questions

GET FREE MEDMIRACLE AIIMS TEST SERIES

- 6 Tests (Including New Pattern Questions As per New Guidelines) & 2 Practice Tests
- For more details check Inner Cover Page—MedMiracle AIIMS Test Series

Acknowledgments

We express sincere gratitude and are thankful to all the Faculties, Subject Specialists, Our Students and the whole Team of MedMiracle for coming together on a single platform & sharing our mission to help & guide each PG Aspirant to fulfill their dream of securing a PG seat.

Recent PG Toppers have gone through and suggested appropriate changes to enhance output through this book.

- Dr Archana Sasi, Rank 1 AIIMS 2017
- Dr Sanchit Kumar, Rank 3 AIIMS 2017
- Dr Umang Arora, Rank 1 AIIMS 2018
- Dr Ayush Goel, Rank 2 AIIMS 2018
- Dr Piyush Aggarwal, Rank 9 AIIMS 2018
- Dr Pavan Gabra, Rank 5 AIIMS 2018
- Dr Komal Gupta, Rank 27 AIIMS May 2019
- Dr Kavan Parikh, Rank 18 NEET PG 2019

Special Thanks to Co-Authors (MedMiracle Mentors)

- Dr Ravi Sharma
- Dr Zainab Vora
- Dr Anivita Aggarwal
- Dr Dipin Sudhakaran
- Dr Armaandeep Singh Aulakh
- Dr Kavan Parikh
- Dr Saurabh Sarda

We as a team will be always grateful for the support provided by leading educationists Dr Gobind Rai Garg, Faculty of Pharmacology; Dr Rebecca James, Faculty of Biochemistry; Dr Sakshi Arora, Faculty of Obstetrics & Gynecology; Dr Rajesh Kaushal, Leading Faculty of Anatomy; Dr Vivek Jain, Faculty of PSM and Dr Sparsh Gupta, Faculty of Pathology in helping us throughout.

Special Thanks to MedMiracle Faculties

1. Dr Subhash Bhukya, MD Anatomy, AIIMS, MedMiracle Faculty of Anatomy
2. Dr Dheeraj, MD Anatomy, AIIMS
3. Dr Navin Gupta, MedMiracle Faculty of Physiology
4. Dr Nilesh Chandra, MedMiracle Faculty of Biochemistry
5. Dr Ashumi, MD Pathology, MedMiracle Faculty of Pathology
6. Dr Anil Sharma, MD Pathology, AIIMS
7. Dr Rachna Rathi, MedMiracle Faculty of Pharmacology
8. Dr Raunak Bir, MD Microbiology, AIIMS MedMiracle Faculty of Microbiology
9. Dr Deepankar, MD Microbiology, AIIMS MedMiracle Faculty of Microbiology

10. Dr Vishwajeet, MedMiracle Faculty of Forensic Medicine
11. Dr Rajanikanta Swain, MD Forensic Medicine, AIIMS, MedMiracle Faculty of Forensic Medicine
12. Dr Manisha Mandal, MD Community Medicine, AIIMS, MedMiracle Faculty of Community Medicine
13. Dr Srikant Kumar, MD Ophthalmology, AIIMS, MedMiracle Faculty of Ophthalmology
14. Dr Meghal Gagrani, MD Ophthalmology, AIIMS, MedMiracle Faculty of Ophthalmology\
15. Dr Gita Srivastava, MS ENT MedMiracle Faculty of ENT
16. Dr Karan Aggarwal, MS ENT, AIIMS
17. Dr Kartik Gupta, MD Medicine, AIIMS, MedMiracle Faculty of Medicine
18. Dr Achintya, MD Medicine, AIIMS, MedMiracle Faculty of Medicine
19. Dr Anand Bhatia, MD Pediatrics, MedMiracle Faculty of Pediatrics
20. Dr Aditya Gupta, MD Pediatrics, AIIMS, MedMiracle Faculty of Pediatrics
21. Dr Neelam Prasad, MD Obs & Gynae, AIIMS, MedMiracle Faculty of OBS & Gynae
22. Dr Amenda Ann Davis, MD Obs & Gynae, AIIMS
23. Dr Bishwanath Tiwari, MedMiracle Faculty of Surgery
24. Dr Aashir Kaul, MS General Surgery, AIIMS, MedMiracle Faculty of Surgery
25. Dr Shivani Kapila, MS General Surgery, AIIMS, MedMiracle Faculty of Surgery
26. Dr Amit Gupta, MD Radiodiagnosis, AIIMS MedMiracle Faculty of Radiology
27. Dr Nikhil Mehta, MD Dermatology, AIIMS, MedMiracle Faculty of Dermatology
28. Dr Sandeep Govil, MD Psychiatry, AIIMS, MedMiracle Faculty of Psychiatry
29. Dr Surabhi Sharma, MD Psychiatry, AIIMS, MedMiracle Faculty of Psychiatry
30. Dr Preeti Yadav, MD Anesthesia, AIIMS, MedMiracle Faculty of Anaesthesia.

A Valuable Drop in The Ocean!

The Idea behind the book AIIMS: The Precise Version stems from the age-old principle of competition exams – "***What has been asked will be asked again***!"

This idea has commonly misinterpreted by various teachers and students alike. It does not mean that the same questions shall be repeated in future exams. Though, old questions are sometimes repeated as it is, they are not sufficient to get you across the line.

With a team of toppers behind this book, we do understand that **it is not the questions but the topics that are repeated**. They were similar in when **Dr Thameem Saif** and **Dr Apurv Mehra** appeared for the exam, when **Dr Vishnu Prasad** and **Dr Akhil Monga** sat for their exams and the list has remained almost the same over the last five years with a few additions. This conclusion has never been challenged by people who have aced the exam. We realized the lacunae in the **exam-oriented revision material available to the students**. An effort has been made to remove redundancy and repetitiveness to make things as crisp as possible, which gives **extra time to the students to revise more and catch up on sleep**. The book flows like a river and allows you to read for long hours without getting bored or tired.

This book aims at providing an insight to the pattern of AIIMS post-graduation entrance exam and at the same time, equipping students with **a topic based quick review** of the most important concepts and facts that have been labeled **high-yield** by our team of toppers.

We aim to reduce the burden on students for preparing their own revision material. This book can act as the base, with students adding their own updates, mnemonics, sticky notes and cheat sheets to it. We firmly believe that it is important to **strengthen your knowledge at the end, rather than looking for more**.

The immense hard work of the authors, co-authors and the contributing faculties and students has made this a **must-read book** for all medical students preparing for the AIIMS postgraduation entrance exam.

An effort has been made to provide you with a glimpse of the **new pattern of questions** that have been announced for the July 2019 session. These questions will test your application but the subject matter remains the same.

This book has been made with an intent to help our juniors as **we understand the turmoil** that hits their lives during this phase. We hope you have a great time reading the book and find it useful in your preparation.

Best Wishes
Team MedMiracle

All Students reading this book are invited to join
MedMiracle Facebook Page
(https://www.facebook.com/medmiracle.in/)
to participate in daily quiz & avail FREE MedMiracle Packs
Also know latest updates/Important Topics/High Yield Questions/ Pearls to stimulus your preparation
Mail All Your Doubts & Queries to drapurv@medmiracle.in
To be directly answered By Dr Apurv Mehra & Dr Thameem Saif along with other Subject Specialists.

Believers Destination
The Dawn of Achievers
Announces
Ortho Dhoom Dhadaka (ODD)

India's Leading Independent Orthopedic Lecture By Dr.Apurv Mehra
ODD is an Orthopedic Lecture for medical students planning for Entrance Exams
AIIMS/NEET/PGI DNB/JIPMER

Ortho Dhoom Dhadaka (ODD) is a program delivering highly verified Orthopedic content to strengthen concepts, add extra edge to your preparation & help you to excel in exams. ODD spreads a ray of hope and helps in dream realization. Thousands of students who have attended ODD across the country have become achievers as a result of highly motivating and enriching interaction. ODD has proudly been honored by toppers in all the exams during 2014-2017.

The First ODD Lecture was organized by Dr Apurv Mehra @ FICCI Auditorium in Delhi on 14thAug 2014.

Conquering all doubts, questions and challenges from the Industry Insiders, ODD @ FICCI Delhi went 'HOUSEFUL' From that point forward there has been no looking back. Rest is all history...

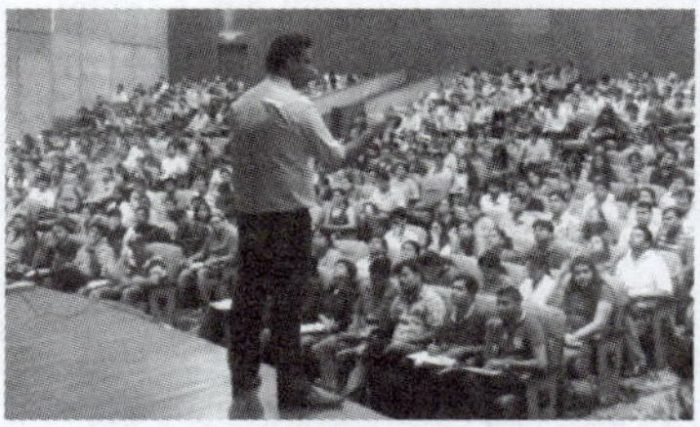

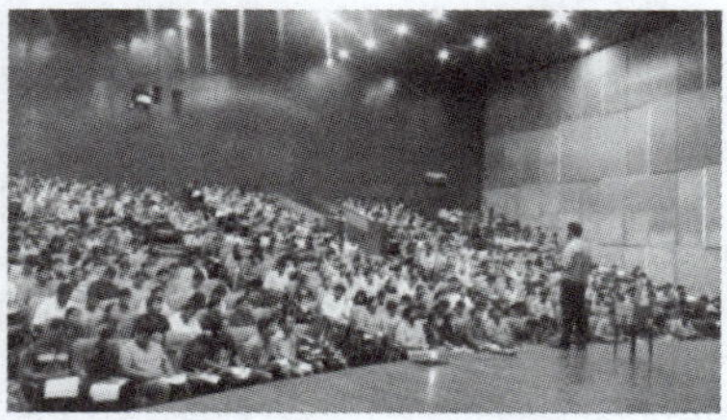

ODD 2.0 SCHEDULE 2020

Register for ODD Get Dr. Apurv Mehra's Orthopedics App FREE
To Register Log Onto: www.drapurv.com

February **Ahmedabad**	**March** **Delhi-1**	**April** **Nagpur**
April **Hyderabad-1**	**May** **Bangalore**	**June** **Aurangabad**
July **Mumbai**	**July** **Delhi-2**	**July** **Hyderabad-2**

For Final dates Log on to www.drapurv.com

Special discounts

• Premium subscribers of Dr Apurv's Orthopedics APP • Group of students
• Toppers • Old ODD Student

Call/Whatsapp To 9999664864 | 8800222009
For Updates Join Facebook Page: Apurv Mehra | Mail Your Queries To drapurv@medmiracle.in

REGD. OFFICE: Vidya Jeevan Ortho Pedics Centre, 28, Vigyan Vihar, Near Yamuma Sports Complex (Gate No. 2)

Timings: Monday To Saturday: 9 am To 9 pm (Sunday Through Appointment Only)
(To Reach us enter Vigyan Vihar on Google Maps)

Dr. Apurv Mehra

For Any Doubt Academic / Nonacademic write to drapurv@medmiracle.in

Dr. Apurv Mehra – The Orthopedic Surgeon

Dr. Apurv Mehra is an Internationally Trained & Experienced Computer Navigation Joint Replacement & Arthroscopy Surgeon

He is an Orthopedic Consultant at Max Institute of Bone & Joint Care at Patparganj, Delhi

Dr. Apurv Mehra is the Founder & Director of Vidya Jeevan Ortho Pedics Centre, Delhi–India's most Trusted Orthopedic Centre as per Leading Clinicians.

He has exceptional academic skills, his clear logical thoughts & approach to complex surgical issues makes him a standout in Knee Arthoplasty & Ligament Reconstructions. His surgical skills & compassionate behavior helps his patients to return back to routine activities & lead a normal life. His clinical skills are exemplary, he achieves good outcomes, and his patients love him.

Dr. Apurv Mehra–Renowned Author, Leading Faculty, Inspirational & Motivational Speaker

Dr. Apurv Mehra is the Leading Faculty of Orthopedics and is recognized Nationally and Internationally as an outstanding teacher, world class scholar & dedicated mentor. Dr. Apurv Mehra is also Co-Founder of MedMiracle–Online Platform to Guide Students Preparing for Medical Entrance Exams. He is best known for his stupendous efforts in teaching, motivating and inspiring budding doctors.

The quality that sets him apart is his unique style of teaching with fun & passion. He is the Author of many International Bestsellers across South East Asia. His books are being appreciated across the globe.

Dr. Apurv Mehra is a youth icon, guide, mentor and role model for aspiring doctors. He is known for his highly inspirational and motivational Speeches.

He has a vision and aims to provide high content resources needed to take students to the next level of education.

Thousands of students have been benefitted by his His Leading Orthopedic Lectures named Ortho Dhoom Dhadaka. His lectures are highly recommended by PG Toppers since Dr. Apurv inspires students to work hard, he builds trust in them and helps them to achieve their goals.

Inspired from his lectures, students not only learn but also follow his advice and guidance in their day to day lives.

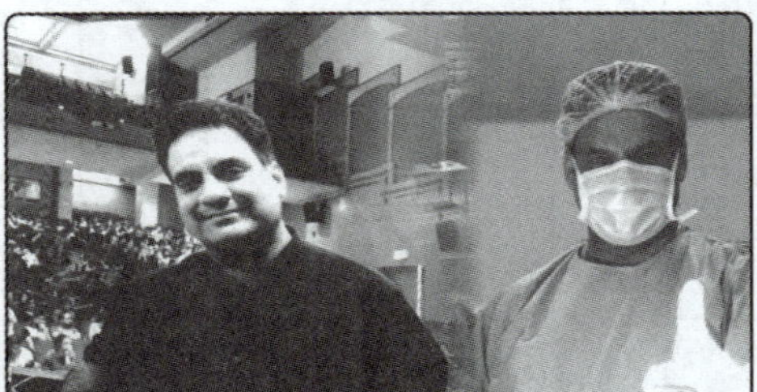

Dr Apurv Mehra's

Vidya Jeevan Orthopedics Super Speciality Centre

Indias Most Trusted Orthopedics Centre For Ethical Practice

28, Vigyan Vihar, Near Yamuna Sports Complex, (Gate No. 2), Delhi-110092.

Centre Timings: Monday to Saturday: 9 am to 9 pm

For Appointments: **8800222008 / 011-41512008**

Dr. Apurv Mehra's Orthopedics App
Food For Your Soul

Most Trusted APP for Orthopedics Preparation

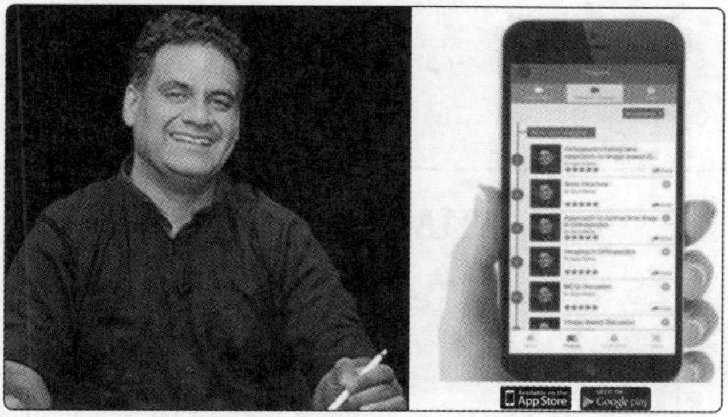

• ✔ PGMEE • ✔ FMGE

- **Chapter Wise Video Lectures According to Significance**
- **Image Based Teaching To Understand Concepts**
- **Test With Video Discussions**
- **Includes The Famous 3 Hours Complete Revision Video Session Added Before Every Exam**
- **Ortho Tests for Practice to Analyze & Evaluate Your Understanding For The Subject.**

New Release • ✔ HINGLISH

Ortho Lectures Now Available in Hindi + English
For Better Understanding Of Concepts

To Subscribe log onto : https://apurvmehra.prepladder.com
To Know More Call on 8800222009 / 9999664864

MedMiracle

Empowers To Excel

An Initiative by Dr. Thameem Saif & Dr. Apurv Mehra

Get FREE MedMiracle AIIMS Test Series

With AIIMS May 2019 Book

✓ 6 Mock Tests ✓ 2 Practice Tests

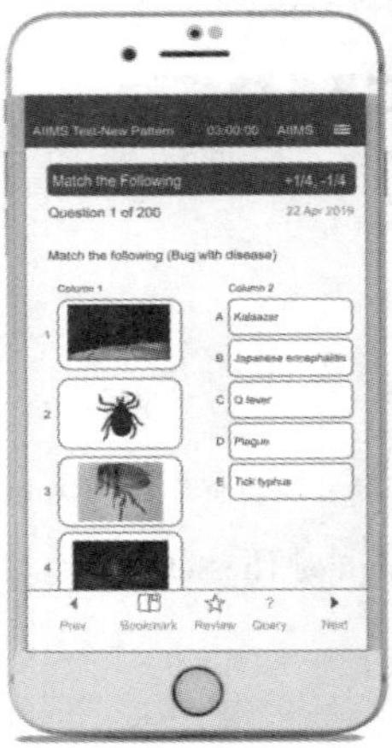

- **Only Online Platform With Exact New Pattern Questions** As Per AIIMS July 2019 Brochure
- All **7 Type Questions** Covering All 19 Subjects
- Authentic Questions With Detailed Explanations & High yielding points
- Prepared By MedMiracle Expert Team
- Detailed Performance Analysis to Identify Your Mistakes
- Know Your Strong Topics & Focus Areas to Improve Your Scores
- Practice Tests on Your Laptop / PC https://medmiracle.in
- Also Available on Medmiracle App Android & iOS

How To Avail Special Offer

Coupon Code

AIIMS + Last 5 Digits of Your Contact No.

For Example:-AIIMS12345

To Apply Code Download Medmiracle App From Google or Apple Playstore
- Click on 'Buy Subscription'
- Click on Test Series & Q. Bank
- Go to << AIIMS Test Series >>
- Type : AIIMS + Last 5 Digits of Your Contact No.
- Click on Submit

For Any Query Call / Whatsapp: 8800222009 / 9999664864

An Initiative by Dr. Apurv Mehra & Dr. Thameem Saif

MedMiracle The App With Only High Yield Content

#1 Bestseller

Complete Pack All 19 Subjects Along with FREE Revision Book

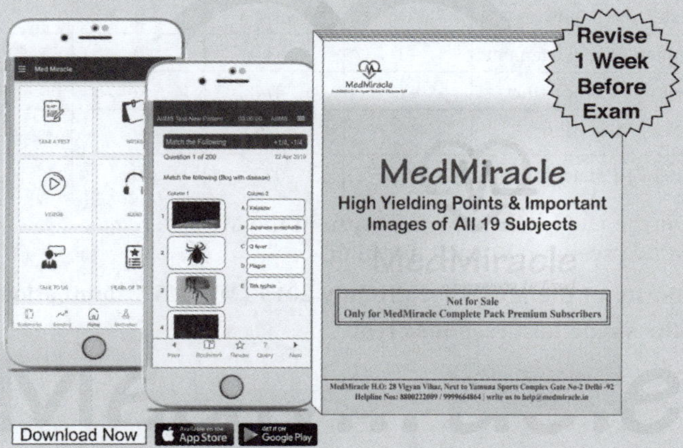

- Concise Notes for Better Understanding
- Practice Only High Yield Questions
- Videos on Important Topics & Previous 3 Years Exam
- Audio Lessons on Volatile Topics
- Pearl of The Day
- Talk to Medmiracle Mentors

Available Subscriptions 3 months | 6 months | 12 months

For Special Offers Call / Whatsapp: 8800222009 / 9999664864

Mail us to help@medmiracle.in

AIIMS Exam New Pattern for July 2019

Type of MCQ	✔	✖	●	○
	Correct	Wrong	For Review	NOT Answered
Single Best Response	+1	–1/3	0	0
Multiple True False*	+1/5	–1/5	0	0
Match the Following*	+1/4	–1/4	0	0
Sequential arrangement	+1	–1	0	0
Multiple Completion	+1	–1/4	0	0
Reason Assertion	+1	–1/4	0	0
Extended Matching**	+1/2	–1/2	0	0

* For the each alternative/response in the MCQ

** If two scenario in each question

Majority of the MCQs for the July 2019 (MD/MS Examination shall be of the single best response type.

Change is the Only Constant in Life!

Dear Friends

AIIMS PGMEE is the most constantly updated exam of the country.

In Latest announcement, AIIMS has introduced 7 different types of MCQs applicable for the upcoming July Session 2019, that is for AIIMS Exam to be held on 5th May 2019.

Now, you don't need to panic, trust me your hard work won't go waste.

In my opinion we need to carefully read and understand the changes announced by AIIMS.

Major Changes

- 7 types of MCQs (including Single best response, Multiple true false, Match the following, Sequential arrangement, Multiple Completion, Assertion-Reason, Extended matching)
- Different marking scheme for each question type
- Time—180 minutes (earlier it was 210 minutes).

Important Footnote (Please read twice)

'Majority of the MCQs for the July 2019 MD/MS Examination shall be of the single best response type'

Now let's understand each one

Type 1: Single Best Answer-Traditional pattern

- Majority of the MCQs for the July 2019 MD/MS Examination shall be of the single best response type – so relax
- **+1 (for correct answer) and-1/3 (for wrong answer). This has been the pattern followed till last AIIMS Nov 2018 Exam**

Example

Q. How many types of MCQs have been introduced in AIIMS PGMEE?

A. 5 B. 6

C. 7 D. 8

Ans. C. 7

Type 2: Multiple True-False

- Common stem followed by 5 statements; each statement has to be marked True/False.
- This pattern resembles PGI questions and can be practiced from previous years' PGI papers.
- +1/5 (for correct answer) and -1/5 (for wrong answer) for each statement.

Example

Q. About AIIMS PGMEE 2019, the following statements are true/ false.

A. Duration of examination is 180 minutes

B. Number of questions is 210

C. 7 types of MCQs will be asked

D. Exam will be in English

E. Exam will be conducted in a single shift on 5th May, 2019.

Ans. A. True B. False (Total number of questions is 200) C. True D. True E. True

Type 3: Match the Following

- Two columns with 4 items in one column which have to be matched with items in second column (which can have more than 4 items) for each alternative.
- Again, *PGI previous years'* have similar questions. With multiple options available for matching, these questions should be relatively easier to attempt.
- +1/4 (for correct answer) and -1/4 (for wrong answer)

Example

Q. Match the Following..?

1. AIIMS Exam Date	a. 200
2. Total questions	b. 5/5/2019
3. Duration (min)	c. 210
4. No of shifts	d. 180
	e. 1
	f. 300

Ans. 1-b, 2-a, 3-d, 4-e

Type 4: Sequential Arrangement

- A list of items that have to be arranged in order as indicated.
- This is a new question type. To tackle this MCQ, basically we need to focus on various pointers to differentiate similar conditions/pathologies and we need to keep in mind how these pathologies compare in different aspects. Beware, this type has a 100% negative marking - Attempt only if you are reasonably confident.
- +1 (for correct answer) and -1 (wrong answer).

Example

Q. Arrange these PG exams in the order of number of questions asked in exam—least number of questions first and maximum number of questions last.

1. AIIMS
2. PGI

3. NEET
4. NIMHANS

Ans. 4-1-2-3

Type 5: Multiple Completion

- 4 statements of which one or more may be correct and SINGLE ANSWER has to be marked according to the given key.
- This type is an easier version of PGI type questions where we have to mark a single answer. Only thing, read the key carefully and then mark.
- +1 (for correct answer) and -1/4 (for wrong answer).

Example

Q. AIIMS new MCQ types include:

A. Multiple true-false
B. Assertion Reason
C. Sequential arrangement
D. Subjective questions

A. a, b, c are correct
B. a and c are correct
C. b and d are correct
D. a, b, c & d are correct

Ans. A. a, b, c are correct

Type 6: Assertion Reason

- This type has been asked in AIIMS-PMT for many years now and has been a trademark for AIIMS MBBS entrance.
- These are tricky questions and we need to correlate basic concepts to tackle these as we need to know how the given two statements are related to each other.
- +1 (for correct answer) -1/4 (for wrong answer).

Example

Assertion: AIIMS is the most sought after institute in the country.
Reason: AIIMS has the latest technology in medical science.

A.	Both Assertion and Reasoning are independently true/correct and Reason is the correct explanation of the Assertion
B.	Both Assertion and Reasoning are independently true/correct and Reason is not the correct explanation of the Assertion
C.	Assertion is independently a true/correct statement but the Reason is independently an incorrect/false statement
D.	Assertion is independently a false/incorrect statement but the Reason is independently a true/correct statement
E.	Both Assertion and Reason are independently a false/incorrect statement

Ans. A. Both Assertion and Reasoning are independently true/correct and Reason is the correct explanation of the Assertion

Type 7: Extended Matching

- Each question has a theme, list of options, main lead question and a number of scenarios. Novel type of question.
- Major issue is the length of the question body since the scenarios are provided as large paragraphs with details about the condition/ pathology. So be sure to read it swiftly and clearly so that you don't lose time. Again, the most important point is to know how similar conditions differ in certain aspects to choose among the given options' list.
- +1/ No of scenarios; -1/ No of scenarios
- +1/2 (for correct answer) -1/2 (for wrong answer) If number of scenario are equal to 2.

Example

Theme-PGMEE

Answer option list:

a. AIIMS

b. NEET

c. PGI

d. NIMHANS

e. JIPMER

Lead Question

For the given scenario, choose the PG exam from the above given list.

Scenario

This exam is one of the toughest in the country. For the most sought after medical college, it is a test of intellect rather than just factual information. The latest MCQ pattern (7 types of questions) makes the exam even more exciting and challenging for the medical aspirants. Identify this institute.

Ans. a. AIIMS

We will come up with more updates about the new AIIMS pattern in future. Keep reading & keep learning.

P.S: For more details, will advise you to check the AIIMS Prospectus https://www.aiimsexams.org/pdf/Eligibility%20%20Method%20of%20 Selection%20July%202019%20.pdf.

Contents

Anatomy

1. Which of the following muscles is not supplied by the nerve marked in the given image?

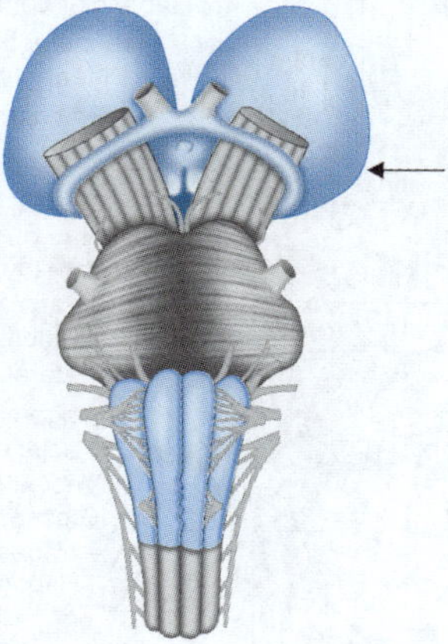

a. Medial rectus
b. Inferior rectus
c. Superior oblique
d. Superior rectus

Ans. c. Superior oblique

The Brainstem

Ventral View

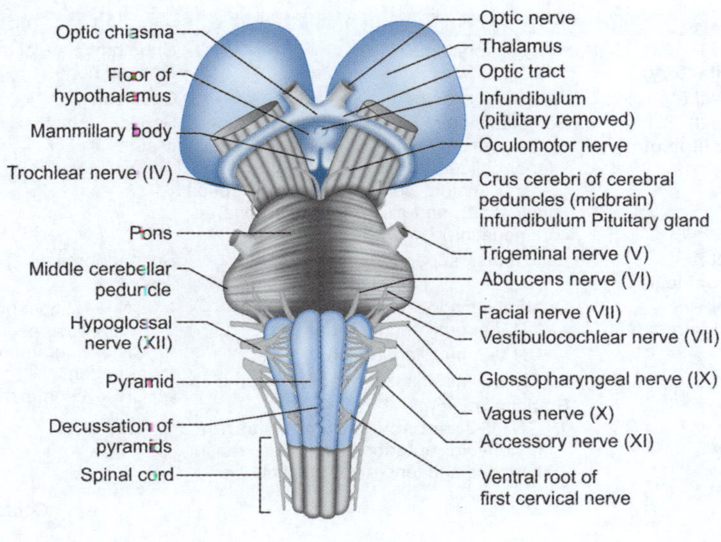

Dorsal View of the Brainstem

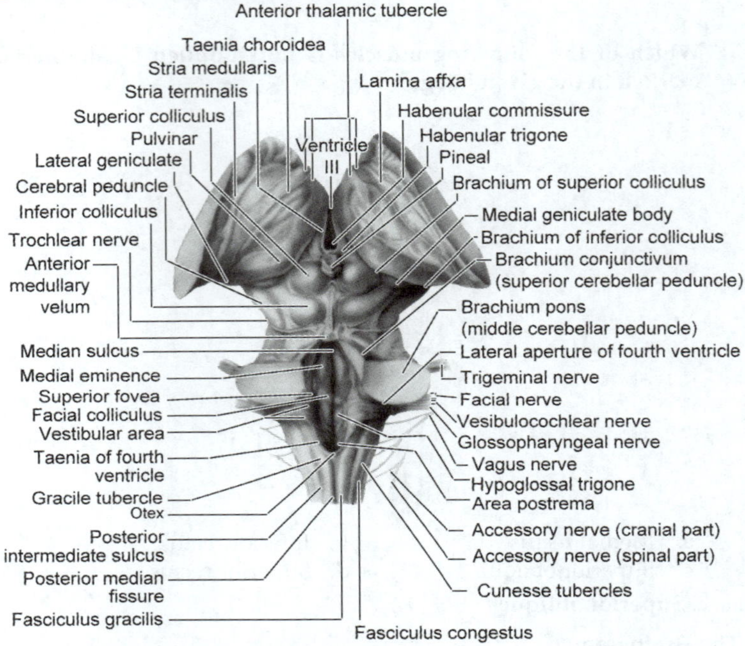

Overview of the Cranial Nerves

CN	Modalities and function	Exit from skull
CN I (olfactory)	Special sensory: smell	Cribriform plate of the ethmoid bone
CN II (optic)	Special sensory: sight	Optic canal
CN III (oculomotor)	➢ Somatic motor: levator palpebrae superioris; superior, medial, and inferior rectus; inferior oblique ➢ Visceral motor: sphincter pupillae (pupil constriction), and ciliary muscles (lens accommodation)	Superior orbital fissure
CN IV (trochlear)	Somatic motor: superior oblique	Superior orbital fissure
CN V (trigeminal)	➢ General sensory: • CN V-1: orbit and forehead • CN V-2: maxillary region • CN V-3: mandibular region, tongue ➢ Branchial motor: • CN V-3: muscles of mastication, mylohyoid, anterior digastricus, tensor tympani, and tensor veli palatini	➢ CN V-1: superior orbital fissure ➢ CN V-2: foramen rotundum ➢ CN V-3: foramen ovale

Contd...

Contd...

CN	Modalities and function	Exit from skull
CN VI (abducens)	Somatic motor: lateral rectus	Superior orbital fissure
CN VII (facial)	➢ General sensory: external acoustic meatus and auricle ➢ Special sensory: anterior two-thirds of tongue ➢ Branchial motor: muscles of facial expression and stylohyoid, posterior digastricus, stapedius. ➢ Visceral motor: lacrimal, submandibular, sublingual, palatal, and nasal glands	Internal acoustic meatus
CN VIII (vestibulocochlear)	Special sensory: hearing, balance, and equilibrium	Internal acoustic meatus
CN IX (glossopharyngeal)	➢ General sensory: posterior third of tongue, oropharynx, tympanic membrane, middle ear, and auditory tube ➢ Special sensory: taste from posterior one-third of tongue ➢ Visceral sensory: carotid sinus (baroreceptor) and carotid body (chemoreceptor) ➢ Branchial motor: stylopharyngeus ➢ Visceral motor: parotid gland	Jugular foramen
CN X (vagus)	➢ General sensory: skin of the posterior ear and external acoustic meatus ➢ Visceral sensory: aortic and carotid bodies (chemoreceptors) and aortic arch (baroreceptor) ➢ Branchial motor: palatal muscles (except tensor tympani); pharyngeal muscles (except stylopharyngeus) and laryngeal muscles. ➢ Visceral motor: heart, smooth muscle, and glands of the respiratory tract, gastrointestinal tube, and viscera of the foregut and midgut	Jugular foramen
CN XI (spinal accessory)	Branchial motor: trapezius and sternocleidomastoid muscles.	Jugular foramen
CN XII (hypoglossal)	Somatic motor: tongue muscles. (except palatoglossus)	Hypoglossal canal

2. Surface marking seen in image corresponds to:

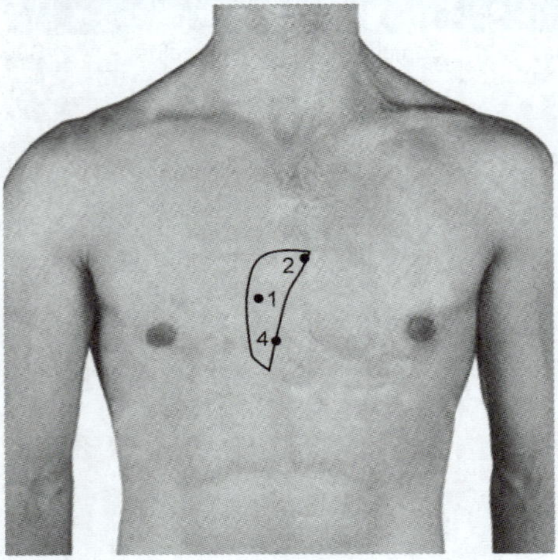

a. Right atrium
b. Thoracic duct
c. Right pulmonary hilum
d. Medial basal segment of right lower lobe

Ans. a. Right atrium

Surface Anatomy of the Heart

The heart rests on the diaphragm and is covered anteriorly by the body of the sternum and the 3rd-6th costal cartilages of both sides. More specifically, the upper limit of the heart reaches as high as the 3rd costal cartilage on the right side of the sternum and the 2nd intercostal space on the left side of the sternum (both 1.2 cm from the sternal border). The right margin of the heart extends from the right 3rd costal cartilage to near the right 6th costal cartilage (at the 6th chondro-sternal junction). The left margin of the heart descends laterally from the 2nd intercostal space to the apex located near the midclavicular line in the 5th intercostal space. The lower margin of the heart extends from the sternal end of the right 6th costal cartilage to the apex in the 5th intercostal space near the midclavicular line (or 9 cm from the midline).

The right border of the heart is formed by the right atrium. The vena cavae enter the heart at the upper and lower ends of the borders. The lower border of the heart is mainly the right ventricle but includes some left ventricle at the apex. It lies at the end of the xiphisternal joint. The lower 4/5 of the left border of the heart is formed by the left ventricle and the upper 1/5 by the left atrium. The upper border is formed by both atria. The superior vena cava enters the heart at its right end, the ascending aorta crosses the middle of the border, the pulmonary trunk bifurcates just above the left end, and the right pulmonary artery runs to the right just above the border.

The chambers of the heart can be marked out by drawing:

The coronary sulcus: Separating the atria and the ventricles from the upper medial end of the 3rd left costal cartilage to the middle of the right 6th chondro-sternal joint.

The anterior interventricular sulcus: from the 3rd left intercostal space 2.5 cm to the left of the midline to a point 1.2 cm medial to the apex.

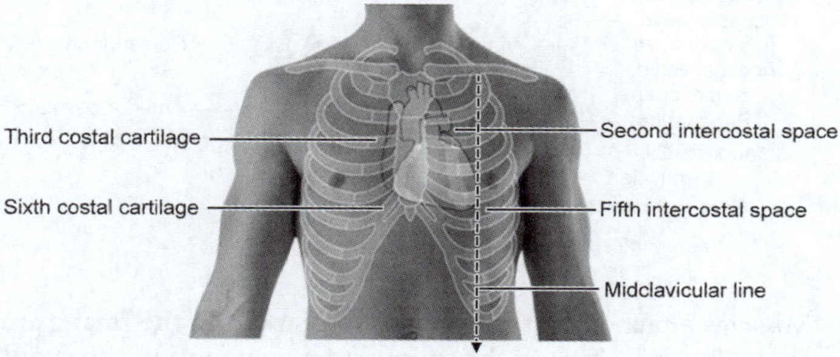

3. Identify the following structures marked in the figure:

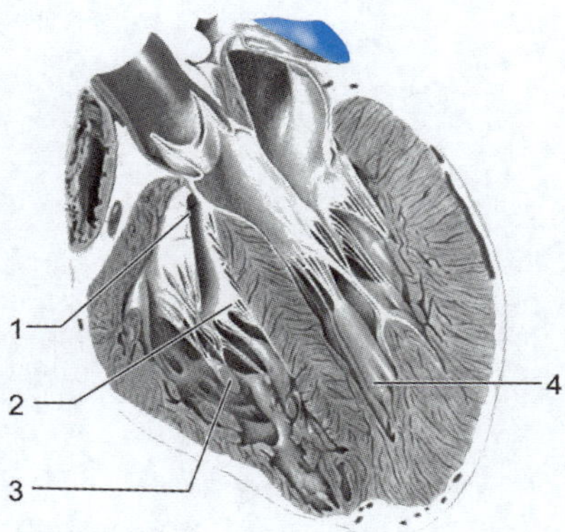

a. Membranous part of interventricular septum
b. Pectinate muscle
c. Anterior papillary muscle of right ventricle
d. Anterior papillary muscle of left ventricle
e. Tendon of Todaro
f. Septal cusp of tricuspid valve

Ans. **1-a, 2-f, 3-c, 4-d**

Internal Structure of the Heart

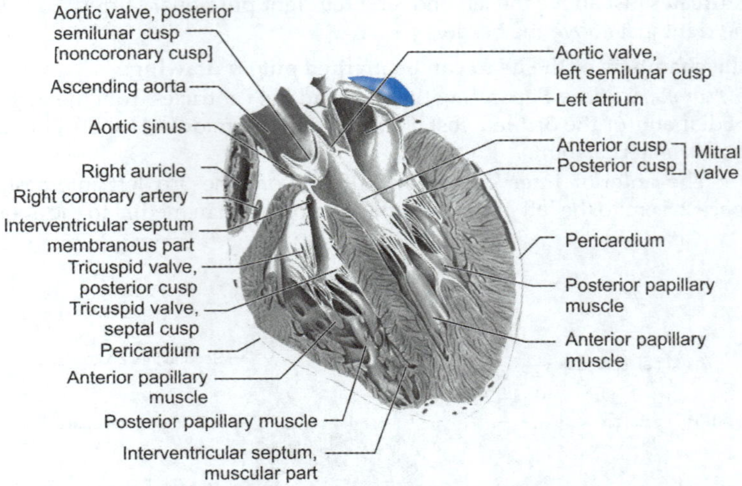

4. Muscles attached on the bony point marked in the image are responsible for which of the following movements of the shoulder joint?

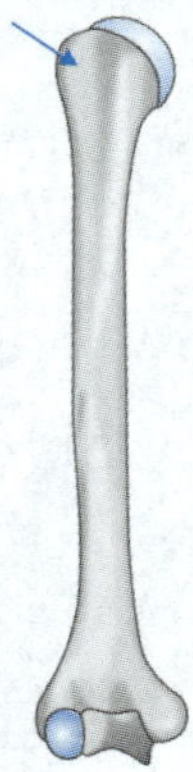

a. Abduction b. Adduction
c. Flexion d. Extension

Ans. **a. Abduction**

Rotator Cuff Muscles

Four of the scapulohumeral muscles (intrinsic shoulder muscles)—supraspinatus, infraspinatus, teres minor, and subscapularis the SITS muscles)—are called rotator cuff muscles because they form a musculotendinous rotator cuff around the glenohumeral joint. All except the supraspinatus are rotators of the humerus; the supraspinatus, besides being part of the rotator cuff, initiates and assists the deltoid in the first 15° of abduction of the arm. The tendons of the SITS muscles blend with and reinforce the fibrous layer of the joint capsule of the glenohumeral joint, thus forming the rotator cuff that protects the joint and gives it stability. The tonic contraction of the contributing muscles holds the relatively large head of the humerus in the small, shallow glenoid cavity of the scapula during arm movements.

Insertions of various muscles of the shoulder joint are shown below:

Posterior view:

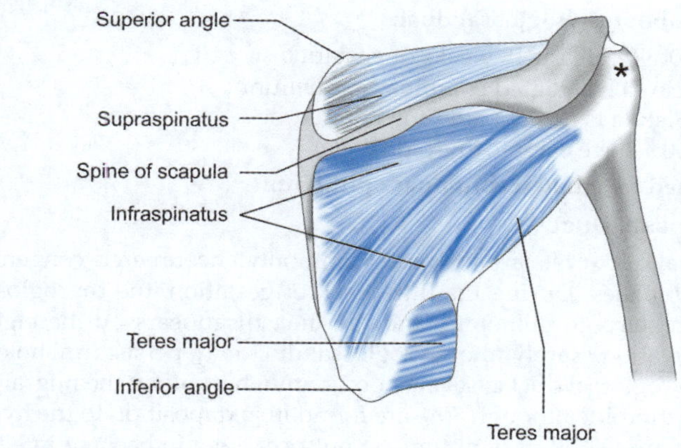

Anterior view:

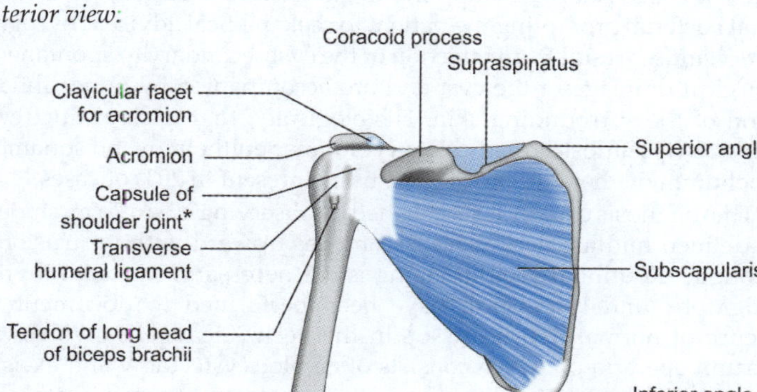

5. Which finger has two dorsal interossei?

a. Middle finger
b. Index finger
c. Thumb
d. Little finger

Ans. a. Middle finger

Muscle	Proximal attachment	Distal attachment	Innervation	Main action
Planter interossei (three muscles)	Planter aspect of medial sides of shafts of metatarsals 3–5	Medial sides of bases of phalanges of 3rd-5th digits	Lateral planter nerve (S2, S3)	Adduct digits 3–5 and flex metatarsophalangeal joints
Dorsal interossei (four muscles)	Adjacent sides of shafts of metatarsals 1–5	1st: Medial side of proximal phalanx of 2nd digit. 2nd-4th: Lateral sides of 2nd–4th digits		Abduct digits 2–4 and flex metatarsophalangeal joints

6. True about thyroglossal duct:

a. Obliterates at 18 weeks of gestation
b. Lined by ciliated columnar epithelium
c. Fistula is formed after infection
d. 40% have ectopic thyroid tissue

Ans. b. Lined by ciliated columnar epithelium

Thyroglossal Duct

Thyroglossal duct cysts are the most commonly encountered congenital cervical anomalies. During the fifth week of gestation, the thyroglossal duct lumen starts to obliterate, and the duct disappears by the eighth week of gestation. Rarely, the thyroglossal duct may persist in whole or in part. Thyroglossal duct cysts may occur anywhere along the migratory path of the thyroid, although 80% are found in juxtaposition to the hyoid bone. They are usually asymptomatic but occasionally become infected by oral bacteria, prompting the patient to seek medical advice. Thyroglossal duct sinuses result from infection of the cyst secondary to spontaneous or surgical drainage of the cyst and are accompanied by minor inflammation of the surrounding skin. Histologically, thyroglossal duct cysts are lined by pseudostratified ciliated columnar epithelium and squamous epithelium, with heterotopic thyroid tissue present in 20% of cases.

The diagnosis usually is established by observing a 1- to 2-cm, smooth, well-defined midline neck mass that moves upward with protrusion of the tongue. Routine thyroid imaging is not necessary, although thyroid scintigraphy and ultrasound have been performed to document the presence of normal thyroid tissue in the neck. Treatment involves the "Sistrunk operation," which consists of en bloc cystectomy and excision of the central hyoid bone to minimize recurrence. Approximately 1% of thyroglossal duct cysts are found to contain cancer, which is usually papillary (85%). The role of total thyroidectomy in this setting is debated, but it is advised in patients with large tumors, particularly if there are additional thyroid nodules and evidence of cyst wall invasion or lymph node metastases. Squamous, Hürthle cell, and anaplastic cancers also have been reported but are rare. Medullary thyroid cancers (MTCs) are, however, not found in thyroglossal duct cysts.

7. After parotidectomy, patient complains of loss of sensation while shaving. Which of the following nerves is likely to be affected?

a. Auriculotemporal nerve
b. Greater auricular nerve
c. Facial nerve
d. Mandibular nerve

Ans. b. Greater auricular nerve

Auriculotemporal nerve is the nerve most commonly injured during parotidectomy. However, loss of sensation during shaving indicates that the person has lost sensation over the angle of mandible, which is supplied by greater auricular nerve.

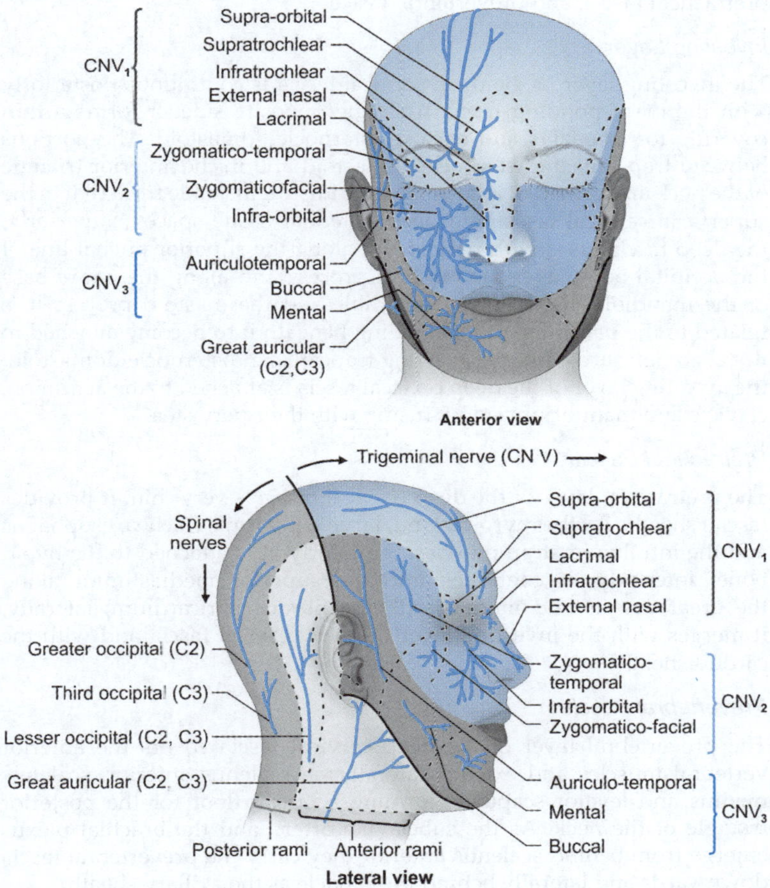

8. Mark the following statements as true or false:

a. Common carotid artery divides at the level of lower border of thyroid cartilage
b. Carotid sheath is formed by the investing layer of deep cervical fascia
c. Ansa cervicalis lies on the posterior wall of carotid sheath
d. Sympathetic chain lies between internal carotid artery and internal jugular vein

Ans. **a-F, b-T, c-F, d-F**

Deep Cervical Fascia

Deep fascia in the neck is conventionally divided into an investing layer, pretracheal fascia, and prevertebral fascia.

Investing Layer

The investing layer of the deep cervical fascia is continuous posteriorly with the corresponding fascia from the opposite side. It forms a thin covering for trapezius and encloses sternocleidomastoid. The portions between trapezius and sternocleidomastoid and in the anterior triangle of the neck are formed of areolar tissue, indistinguishable from that in the superficial cervical fascia and deep potential tissue spaces. Superiorly, the deep fascia fuses with periosteum along the superior nuchal line of the occipital bone, over the mastoid process and along the entire base of the mandible. Between the mandible and the mastoid process it is related to the parotid gland, extending beneath it to become attached to the zygomatic arch. Inferiorly, along trapezius and sternocleidomastoid, the investing layer of the deep cervical fascia is attached to the acromion, clavicle and manubrium sterni, fusing with their periostea.

Pretracheal Fascia

The pretracheal layer of the deep cervical fascia is very thin. It provides fascial sheaths for the thyroid gland, larynx, pharynx, trachea, esophagus and the infrahyoid strap muscles. Superiorly, it is attached to the hyoid bone; inferiorly, it continues into the superior mediastinum along the great vessels and merges with the fibrous pericardium; laterally, it merges with the investing layer of deep cervical fascia and with the carotid sheath.

Prevertebral Fascia

The prevertebral layer of the deep cervical fascia covers the anterior vertebral muscles and extends laterally on scalenus anterior, scalenus medius and levator scapulae, forming a fascial floor for the posterior triangle of the neck. As the subclavian artery and the brachial plexus emerge from behind scalenus anterior they carry the prevertebral fascia downwards and laterally behind the clavicle as the axillary sheath.

The prevertebral fascia is particularly prominent in front of the vertebral column, where there may be two distinct layers of fascia. The space created by the splitting of the anterior prevertebral fascia, the danger space, is a part of the prevertebral space. Superiorly it is attached to the base of the skull. Inferiorly it descends in front of longus colli into the superior mediastinum, where it blends with the anterior longitudinal ligament. Anteriorly the prevertebral fascia is separated from the pharynx and its covering buccopharyngeal fascia by a loose areolar zone, the retropharyngeal space. Laterally this loose tissue connects the prevertebral fascia to the carotid sheath and the fascia on the deep surface of sternocleidomastoid.

Carotid Sheath

The carotid sheath is a condensation of deep cervical fascia around the common carotid artery, which divides at the level of upper border of thyroid cartilage into external and internal carotid arteries, the internal jugular vein, the vagus nerve and the constituents of the ansa cervicalis, along its anterior aspect. It is thicker around the arteries than the vein, an arrangement that allows the vein to expand. Peripherally the carotid sheath is connected to adjacent fascial layers by loose areolar tissue. The sympathetic chain lies posterior to the contents of the carotid sheath.

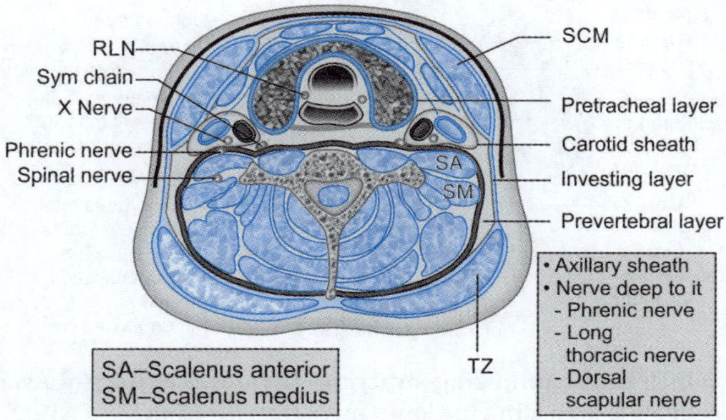

9. Regarding levator ani all are true *except*:

a. Attached to pelvic brim
b. Converges downward and medially
c. Consists of pubococcygeus and iliococcygeus
d. Supports pelvic viscera

Ans. a. Attached to pelvic brim

Levator Ani

The pelvic diaphragm is a muscular partition formed by the levator ani and coccygei, with which may be included by the parietal pelvic fascia on their upper and lower aspects. This diaphragm separates the pelvic cavity from the perineal region. The muscles of the pelvic diaphragm extend from the lateral pelvic walls downward and medially to fuse with each other and are inserted into the terminal portions of the urethra, vagina, and anus.

Levator ani muscle (Pubococcygeus, Iliococcygeus and puborectalis): These muscles and their investing fascia are critical to maintaining support for the vagina and bladder. Rupture or stretch of this support system following pregnancy or childbirth is one of the major causes of pelvic support defects (hernias) and the attendant problems of urinary incontinence and fecal retention. It is to the tendinous arch (arcus tendineus) that some transabdominal approaches to the treatment of cysto-urethroceles provide anchorage or reattachment. The levator sling is also the plate on which pessaries must rest to provide mechanical support to prolapsing pelvic organs.

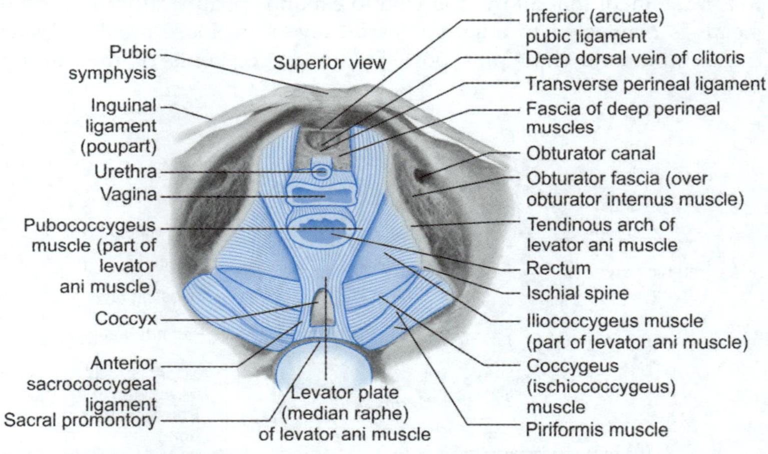

10. Which of the following structures divides the liver into various segments according to Couinaud's classification?

a. Hepatic vein
b. Bile duct
c. Portal vein
d. Porta hepatis

Ans. c. Portal vein

Functional Anatomical Divisions of Liver

Current understanding of the functional anatomy of the liver is based on Couinaud's division of the liver into eight (subsequently nine) functional segments, based upon the distribution of portal venous branches and the location of the hepatic veins in the parenchyma (Couinaud). Further understanding of the intrahepatic biliary anatomy, especially of the right ductal system, was enhanced by contributions from Hjortsjo and Healey & Schroy using the biliary system as the main guide for division of the liver. The liver is divided into four portal sectors by the four main branches of the portal vein. These are right lateral, right medial, left medial and left lateral (sometimes the term posterior is used in place of lateral and anterior in place of medial). The three main hepatic veins lie between these sectors as intersectorial veins. These intersectoral planes are also called portal fissures (scissures). The fissures containing portal pedicles are called hepatic fissures. Each sector is sub-divided into segments (usually two) based on their supply by tertiary divisions of the vascular biliary sheaths.

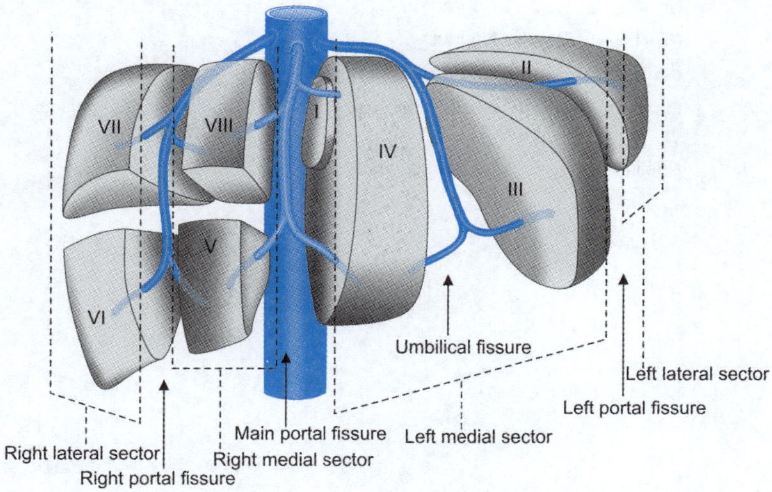

11. Which of the following is not an intermediate filament?

a. Vimentin
b. Cytokeratin
c. Desmin
d. Tubulin

Ans. d. Tubulin

Intermediate filaments are stable cytoskeletal components which confer increased mechanical stability to cell structure, and are made up of different protein subunits in different cell types.

Major classes of intermediate filament proteins are summarized below:

Class	Protein	Cell distribution	Disease involvement
I	Acidic cytokeratin	Epithelial cells	Certain skin-blistering disorders
II	Basic cytokeratin	Epithelial cells	Keratoderma; corneal dystrophy
III	Desmin	Muscle cells	Myopathies
	Synemin	Muscle cells	
	GFAP	Astrocytes (less in other glial cells)	Alexander disease
	Peripherin	Neurons	
	Vimentin	Mesenchymal cells	
IV	NF-L	Neurons	
	NF-M	Neurons	
	NF-H	Neurons	
	α-Internexin	Embryonic neurons	
V	Lamins	Nuclei of all cells	Cardiomyopathy; muscular dystrophies; progeria
VI	Nestin	Neural stem cells	

Physiology

1. Identify the sequence in which clotting factors are activated in intrinsic coagulation pathway:

a. XII
b. XI
c. X
d. IX

Ans. **a-XII, b-XI, d-IX, c-X**

Coagulation Cascade

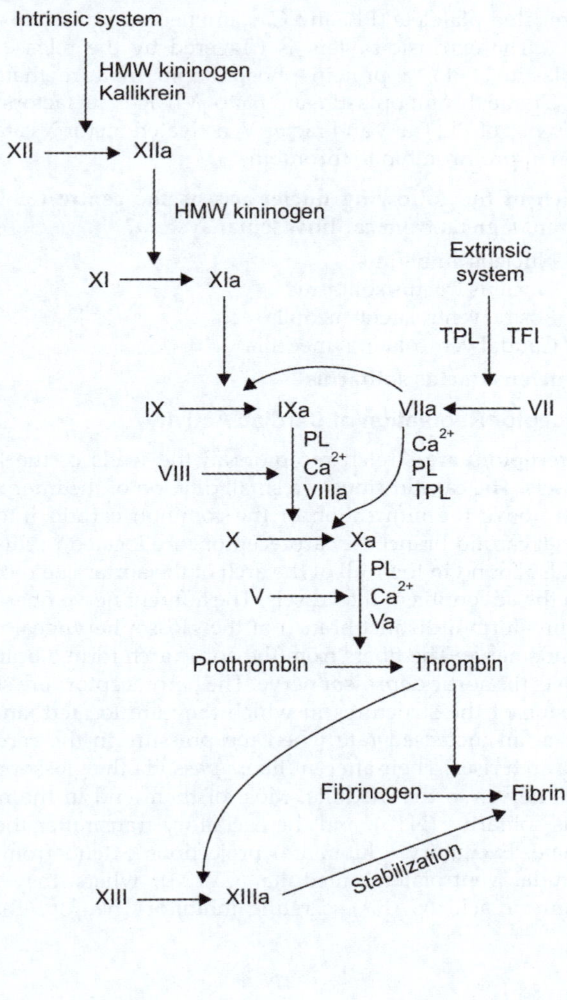

Clotting involves aggregation of platelets followed by formation of fibrin. Fibrin is derived from fibrinogen with the help of thrombin. Thrombin is formed by activation of prothrombin by factor X and V. Factor X can be activated by either of two systems, known as intrinsic and extrinsic. The initial reaction in the intrinsic system is conversion of inactive factor XII to active factor XII (XIIa). This activation, which is catalyzed by high-molecular-weight kininogen and kallikrein, can be brought about *in vitro* by exposing the blood to glass, or *in vivo* by collagen fibers underlying the endothelium. Active factor XII then activates factor XI, and active factor XI activates factor IX. Activated factor IX forms a complex with active factor VIII, which is activated when it is separated from von Willebrand factor. The complex of IXa and VIIIa activate factor X. Phospholipids from aggregated platelets (PL) and Ca^{2+} are necessary for full activation of factor X. The extrinsic system is triggered by the release of tissue thromboplastin (TPL), a protein–phospholipid mixture that activates factor VII. Tissue thromboplastin and factor VII activate factors IX and X. In the presence of PL, Ca^{2+}, and factor V, activated factor X catalyzes the conversion of prothrombin to thrombin.

2. Which of the following nuclei acts as the centre for receiving afferent signals from cardiovascular system?

a. Nucleus ambiguus
b. Nucleus tractus solitarius
c. Rostral ventrolateral medulla
d. Caudal ventrolateral medulla

Ans. **b. Nucleus tractus solitarius**

Baroreceptor Regulation of Cardiac Activity

The baroreceptors are stretch receptors in the walls of the heart and blood vessels. The carotid sinus is a small dilation of the internal carotid artery just above the bifurcation of the common carotid into external and internal carotid branches. Baroreceptors are located in this dilation. They are also found in the wall of the arch of the aorta. The receptors are located in the adventitia of the vessels. The afferent nerve fibers from the carotid sinus form a distinct branch of the glossopharyngeal nerve, the carotid sinus nerve. The fibers from the aortic arch form a branch of the vagus nerve, the aortic depressor nerve. The baroreceptors are stimulated by distension of the structures in which they are located, and so they discharge at an increased rate when the pressure in the carotid sinus and aortic arch rises. Their afferent fibers pass via the glossopharyngeal and vagus nerves to the medulla. Most of them end in the nucleus of the tractus solitarius (NTS), and the excitatory transmitter they secrete is glutamate. Excitatory (glutamate) projections extend from the NTS to the caudal ventrolateral medulla (CVLM), where they stimulate γ-aminobutyric acid (GABA)-secreting inhibitory neurons that project to the RVLM. Excitatory projections also extend from the NTS to the vagal motor neurons in the nucleus ambiguus and dorsal motor nucleus. Thus, increased baroreceptor discharge inhibits the tonic discharge of sympathetic nerves and excites the vagal innervation of the heart. These neural changes produce vasodilation, venodilation, hypotension, bradycardia, and a decrease in cardiac output.

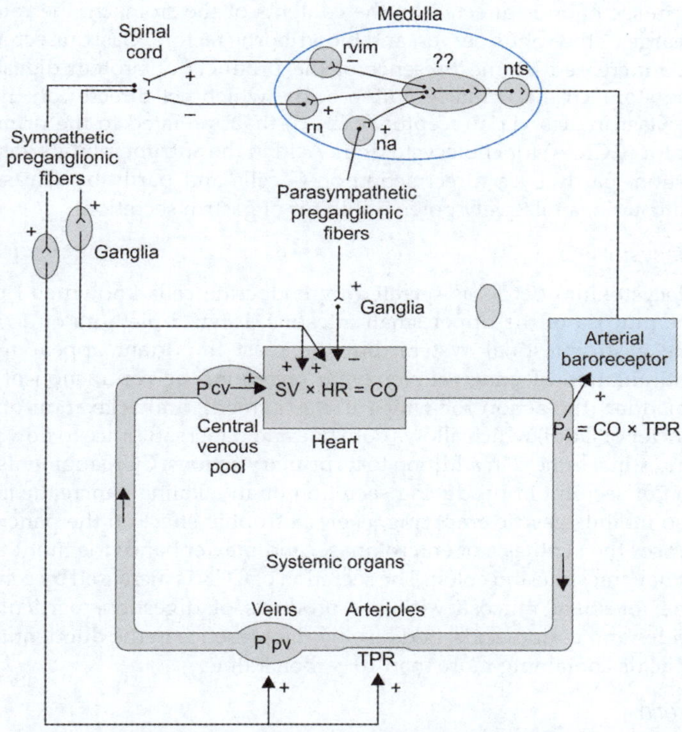

Components of the arterial baroreceptor reflex pathway.

Abbreviation: nts, nucleus tractus solitarius; rvlm, rostral ventrolateral medullary group; rn, raphé nucleus; na, nucleus ambiguus; ??, incompletely mapped integration pathways that may also involve structures outside the medulla.

3. Which of the following peptides do not act on pancreas?

a. Secretin
b. CCK
c. Gastrin
d. GIP

Ans. c. Gastrin

Gastrointestinal Peptides

Gastrin

Gastrin is produced by cells called G cells in the antral portion of the gastric mucosa. The principal physiologic actions of gastrin are stimulation of gastric acid and pepsin secretion and stimulation of the growth of the mucosa of the stomach and small and large intestines (trophic action). Gastrin secretion is affected by the contents of the stomach, the rate of discharge of the vagus nerves, and blood-borne factors. Gastrin secretion is also increased by the presence of the products of protein digestion in the stomach, particularly amino acids, which act directly on the G cells. Gastrin acts via a receptor (CCK-B) that is related to the primary receptor (CCK-A) for cholecystokinin. Acid in the antrum inhibits gastrin secretion, partly by a direct action on G cells and partly by release of somatostatin, a relatively potent inhibitor of gastrin secretion.

Cholecystokinin

Cholecystokinin (CCK) is secreted by endocrine cells known as I cells in the mucosa of the upper small intestine. It has a plethora of actions in the gastrointestinal system, but the most important appear to be the stimulation of pancreatic enzyme secretion; the contraction of the gallbladder (the action for which it was named); and relaxation of the sphincter of Oddi, which allows both bile and pancreatic juice to flow into the intestinal lumen. In addition to its primary actions, CCK augments the action of secretin in producing secretion of an alkaline pancreatic juice. It also inhibits gastric emptying, exerts a trophic effect on the pancreas, increases the synthesis of enterokinase, and may enhance the motility of the small intestine and colon. The secretion of CCK is increased by contact of the intestinal mucosa with the products of digestion, particularly peptides and amino acids, and also by the presence in the duodenum of fatty acids containing more than 10 carbon atoms.

Secretin

Secretin is secreted by S cells that are located deep in the glands of the mucosa of the upper portion of the small intestine. Secretin increases the secretion of bicarbonate by the duct cells of the pancreas and biliary tract. It thus causes the secretion of a watery, alkaline pancreatic juice. It also augments the action of CCK in producing pancreatic secretion of digestive enzymes. It decreases gastric acid secretion and may cause contraction of the pyloric sphincter. The secretion of secretin is increased by the products of protein digestion and by acid bathing the mucosa of the upper small intestine. Secretin causes alkaline pancreatic juice to flood into the duodenum, neutralizing the acid from the stomach and thus inhibiting further secretion of the hormone.

GIP

Gastric inhibitory polypeptide (GIP) is produced by K cells in the mucosa of the duodenum and jejunum. Its secretion is stimulated by glucose and fat in the duodenum. GIP stimulates insulin secretion at physiological levels. For this reason, it is often called glucose-dependent insulinotropic peptide.

VIP

Vasoactive intestinal polypeptide (VIP) is found in nerves in the gastrointestinal tract and thus is not itself a hormone, despite its similarities to secretin. In the intestine, it markedly stimulates intestinal secretion of electrolytes and hence of water. Its other actions include relaxation of intestinal smooth muscle, including sphincters; dilation of peripheral blood vessels; and inhibition of gastric acid secretion.

Motilin

Motilin is secreted by enterochromaffin cells and Mo cells in the stomach, small intestine, and colon. It acts on G-protein-coupled receptors on enteric neurons in the duodenum and colon and produces contraction of smooth muscle in the stomach and intestines in the period between meals.

Somatostatin

Somatostatin, the growth hormone—inhibiting hormone originally isolated from the hypothalamus, is secreted as a paracrine by D cells in the pancreatic islets and by similar D cells in the gastrointestinal mucosa. Somatostatin inhibits the secretion of gastrin, VIP, GIP, secretin, and motilin. Its secretion is stimulated by acid in the lumen, and it acts in a paracrine fashion to mediate the inhibition of gastrin secretion produced by acid. It also inhibits pancreatic exocrine secretion; gastric acid secretion and motility; gallbladder contraction; and the absorption of glucose, amino acids, and triglycerides.

4. Which of the following does Golgi tendon organ detect?

a. Muscle tension
b. Dynamic muscle length
c. Static muscle length
d. Muscle action

Ans. a. Muscle tension

Golgi Tendon Organ

- It is an encapsulated receptor, located within the tendon of a muscle.
- Each Golgi tendon organ is connected to 10–15 muscle fibers.

- Golgi tendon organ functions as a transducer in a feedback circuit that regulates muscle force in a fashion analogous to the spindle feedback circuit that regulates muscle length.
- Unlike muscle spindles, Golgi tendon organs are in series with the muscle fibers, so they are stimulated by both passive stretch and active contraction of muscle.
- It is important to note that spindle detects muscle length and changes in muscle length, whereas Golgi tendon detects muscle tension.
- So it is stimulated when muscle fiber is tensed by contracting or stretching muscle.

5. I-125 labelled albumin is used to measure:

a. Extracellular fluid
b. Intracellular fluid
c. Plasma
d. Interstitial fluid

Ans. c. Plasma

Body Fluid Composition

- Approximately 60% of total body weight in adults is composed of water.

The distribution of water in various compartments of the body is summarized in the following diagram.

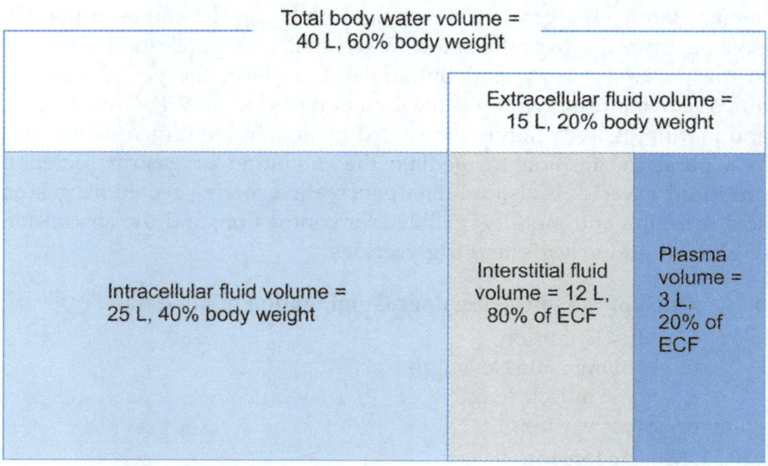

- Most of the fluids are calculated directly from dilution methods, except for ICF and interstitial fluids. Both of these are calculated indirectly by calculating other body fluids.

- ICF = Total body water volume – ECF volume
- Interstitial fluid = ECF volume – Plasma volume

The indicators used for ascertaining fluid volume in various compartments are:

- Total body water volume
  - Deuterium oxide
  - Tritium oxide, Aminopyrine, Antipyrine
- Extracellular fluid volume
  - Inulin
  - 22Na, 125I-iothalamate, thiosulfate
- Plasma volume
  - Evans blue
  - Serum albumin labeled with radioactive iodine (I-125)
- Blood volume - 51Cr-labeled RBCs

6. Which of the following hormones act on intracellular receptor?

a. Thyroxine
b. Insulin
c. Glucagon
d. Calcitonin

Ans. **a. Thyroxine**

Types of hormonal receptors

Bind to intracellular receptor	Bind to cell surface receptor second messenger			
Cytoplasmic receptors Glucocorticoids Mineralocorticoids Androgens, estrogen and progestins Vitamin D3 (1,25-$(OH)_2$ D_3)	c-AMP ➢ Calcitonin ➢ Glucagon ➢ LH & FSH ➢ Norepinephrine	c-GMP ➢ ANF ➢ NO	Ca^{2+}/phosphatidyl inositol ➢ α1 adrenergic ➢ Angiotensin II ➢ Oxytocin ➢ GnRH	Kinase / phosphatase ➢ Insulin ➢ GH ➢ EGF, FGF ➢ IGF I & II
Nuclear receptors ➢ Thyroid hormones ➢ Retinoic acid	➢ HCG ➢ ADH ➢ CRH ➢ PTH ➢ TSH		➢ Substance P ➢ Gastrin ➢ Cholecystokinin ➢ Muscarinic (acetylcholine) ➢ Vasopressin ➢ TRH	➢ Nerve growth factor (NGF) ➢ PDGF ➢ Erythropoietin ➢ Prolactin ➢ Adiponectin and leptin

7. Which of the following factors influence the GFR?

a. Afferent arteriolar resistance
b. Efferent arteriolar resistance
c. Arterial pressure
d. Mesangial contraction
e. None

Ans. **a-T, b-T, c-T, d-T**

Glomerular Filtration Rate (GFR)

- GFR is the rate at which plasma ultrafiltrate is formed by filtration through the glomerulus.

Factors Affecting GFR

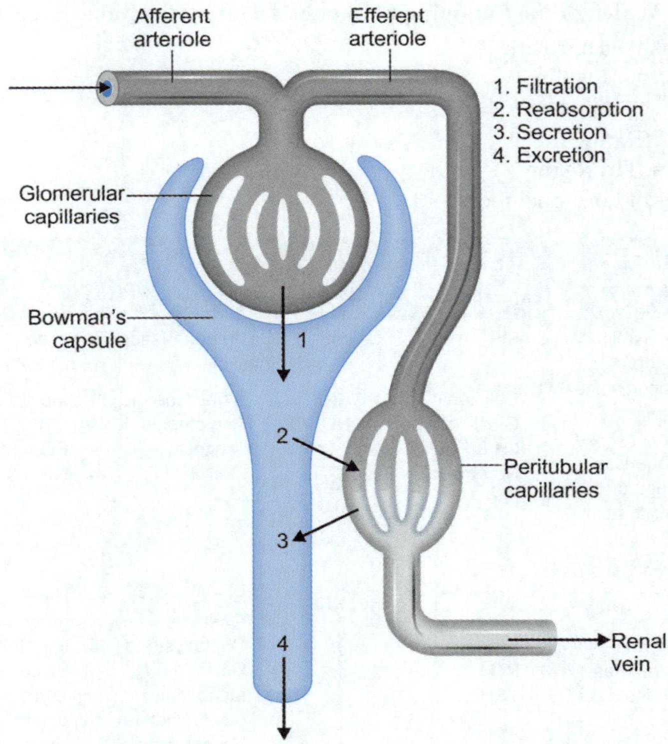

It can be seen from the diagram that glomerular filtration is dependent on several factors; the exact relation can be stated thus:

GF = Kf net filtration pressure, where Kf is the glomerular capillary filtration coefficient.

GF = Kf (Capillary hydrostatic pressure – glomerular hydrostatic pressure + glomerular oncotic pressure – capillary oncotic pressure)

Glomerular oncotic pressure is zero normally since proteins are not filtered.

If efferent arteriole is constricted, the capillary hydrostatic pressure increases. This causes **the glomerular filtration to increase**. Increase in GFR causes an increase in the amount of fluid in the glomerulus, causing an **increase in the glomerular hydrostatic pressure.** Since glomerular filtration increases, more water escapes out of the glomerular capillaries, making the remaining blood more concentrated. Hence the **peritubular oncotic pressure increases**. Also, constriction of efferent arteriole causes a **decrease in both total renal blood flow, as well as a relative blood flow to peritubular capillaries** due to increased filtering at the glomerular level. Mesangial contraction is produced by various peptides decreases the filtration rate.

8. Arrange the following in correct sequence of spermatogenesis:

a. Spermatogonia
b. Spermatocyte
c. Spermatids
d. Spermatozoa

Ans. a-Spermatogonia, b-Spermatocyte, c-Spermatids, d-Spermatozoa

Spermatogenesis

Spermatogonia, the primitive germ cells next to the basal lamina of the seminiferous tubules, mature into primary spermatocytes. This process begins during adolescence. The primary spermatocytes undergo meiotic division, reducing the number of chromosomes. In this two-stage process, they divide into secondary spermatocytes and then into spermatids, which contain the haploid number of 23 chromosomes. The spermatids mature into spermatozoa (sperm). As a single spermatogonium divides and matures, its descendants remain tied together by cytoplasmic bridges until the late spermatid stage. This arrangement helps ensure synchrony of the differentiation of each clone of germ cells. The estimated number of spermatids formed from a single spermatogonium is 512. The formation of a mature spermatozoa from a primitive germ cell by spermatogenesis in humans spans approximately 74 days.

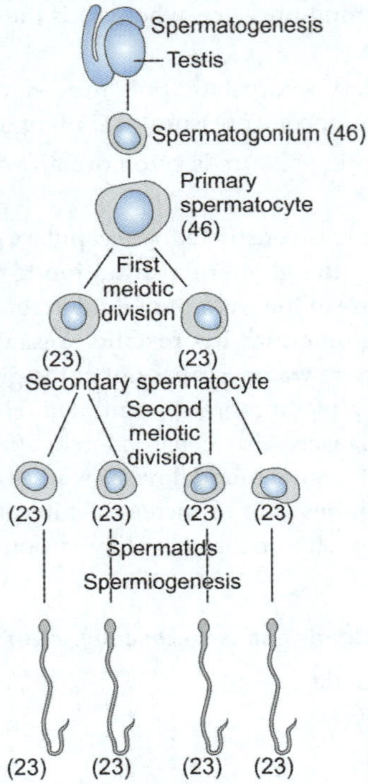

9. Anatomical dead space measured by:

a. Bohler's method
b. Xenon dilution technique
c. Spirometry
d. Single breath nitrogen test

Ans. d. Single breath nitrogen test

Dead Space

- The gas present within the airways is not available for gaseous exchange with the pulmonary vasculature. This volume of gases is known as the anatomical dead space.
- With each expiration, first 150 mL expired is gas that occupied dead space, and only last 350 mL is gas from alveoli.
- Anatomic dead space can be measured by analysis of single-breath N_2 curves.
- From mid-inspiration, subject takes as deep a breath as possible of pure O_2, then exhales steadily while the N_2 content of expired gas is continuously measured.

- Initial gas exhaled (phase I) is the gas that filled the dead space and that consequently contains no N_2. This is followed by a mixture of dead space and alveolar gas (phase II) and then by alveolar gas (phase III).

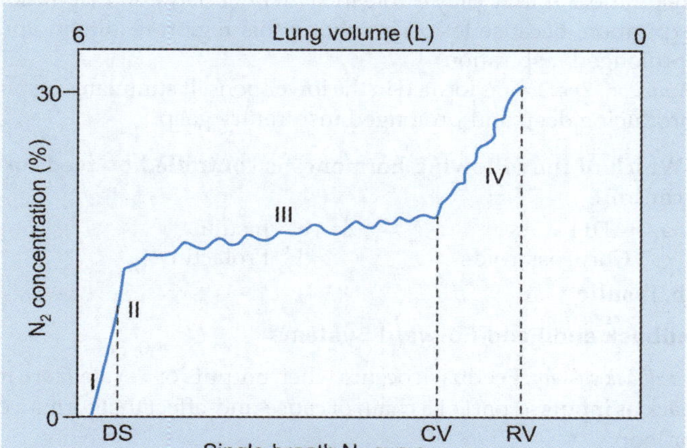

Single-breath N_2 curve

- Volume of dead space is the volume of the gas expired from peak inspiration to the mid portion of phase II.
- Phase III of single-breath N_2 curve terminates at closing volume (CV) and is followed by phase IV, during which N_2 content of expired gas is increased.

10. Which of the following is the centre of rhythm generation of respiration?

a. Prebotzinger complex
b. Dorsal medulla
c. Ventral medulla
d. Pneumotaxic centre

Ans. a. Prebotzinger complex

Regulation of Respiration

Various brainstem centres involved in regulation of respiration are listed below:

- *Dorsal respiratory group (DRG)*: It fires rhythmically during inspiration and hence is primarily responsible for maintaining inspiration. It also serves as initial processing centre for afferent inputs from peripheral chemoreceptors and baroreceptors
- *Ventral respiratory group (VRG)*: It remains inactive during normal breathing and is primarily responsible for active expiration during forceful breathing.

- *Prebotzinger complex*: Pacemaker for initiating spontaneous rhythmic respiration
- *Pneumotaxic center*: It is located in the pons and is active during inspiration. It may play a role in switching between inspiration and expiration, because lesion involving this region results in apneusis (prolonged inspiration)
- *Apneustic center*: It is located in the lower pons. It stimulates inspiration producing deep and prolonged inspiratory gasp.

11. Which of the following hormones is controlled by feed forward control?

a. ADH b. Insulin
c. Corticosteroids d. Prolactin

Ans. b. Insulin

Feedback and Feed-Forward Systems

1. *Feedback system*: Feedback occurs when outputs of a system are routed back as inputs as part of a chain of cause-and-effect that forms a circuit or loop.

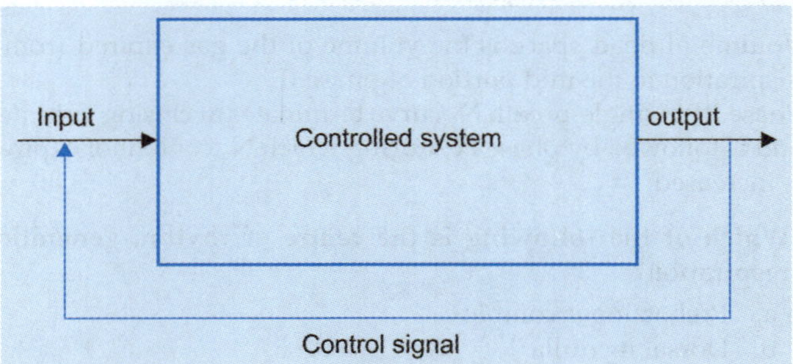

- Positive feedback
  - Estrogen control of GnRH release at ovulation
- Negative feedback
  - Blood pressure
  - Plasma osmolarity
  - Plasma CO_2 and pH
  - Endocrine gland secretion

2. *Feed-forward system*: In this system, the disturbances are measured and accounted for before they have time to affect the system. That is, anticipatory changes are made before the disturbance causes any change in the output. This system has some prerequisites, like how the system works and measurement of the changes caused by the feedforward on the output, since the control variable adjustment is not error-based.

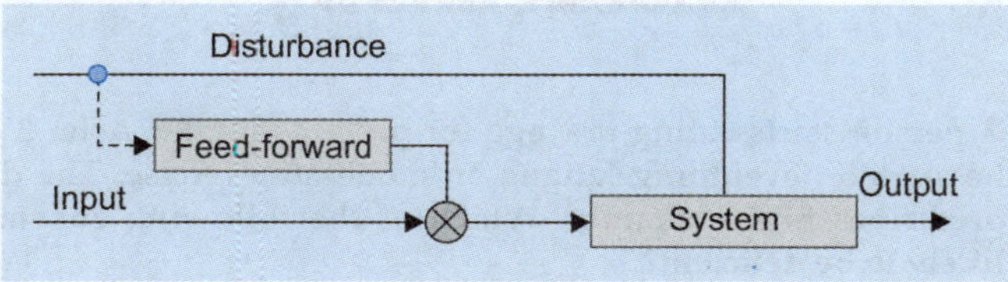

This type of control is anticipatory control. Secretion of insulin by incretins (GIP, GLP) can be considered as feed-forward in nature.

Biochemistry

1. A person starts eating raw egg for proteins intake. After 3 days, he started developing fatigue on moderate exercise. The doctor prescribes him a vitamin. Which of the following enzymes is likely to be deficient?

a. Pyruvate carboxylase
b. PEPCK
c. Glucose 6 phosphatase
d. Glycogen phosphorylase

Ans. **a. Pyruvate carboxylase**

Biotin

- Biotin acts as cofactor in a number of carboxylation reactions involving- acetyl-CoA carboxylase, pyruvate carboxylase, propionyl-CoA carboxylase, and methylcrotonyl-CoA carboxylase.
- It is also involved in catabolism of certain amino acids (leucine) and gene regulation by histone biotinylation.

Biotin functions to transfer carbon dioxide in reactions

- *Pyruvate carboxylase*: Pyruvate is converted to oxaloacetate in gluconeogenesis
- *Acetyl-CoA carboxylase*: Acetyl-CoA is converted to malonyl-CoA in fatty acid synthesis
- *Propionyl-CoA carboxylase*: Propionyl-CoA is converted to methylmalonyl-CoA in gluconeogenesis
- *Methylmalonyl CoA carboxyl transferase*: Propionic acid synthesis in bacteria
- *Methylcrotonyl-CoA carboxylase*: Leucine catabolism

Source:

- Meat, soya beans, yeast and egg yolks
- Egg white contains protein avidin, which strongly binds to biotin, reducing its bioavailability.

Deficiency:

- Biotin deficiency due to low dietary intake is rare (deficiency is due to inborn errors of metabolism)
- Mental changes (depression, hallucinations), paresthesia, anorexia and nausea.
- A scaling, seborrheic, erythematous rash around eyes, nose, mouth and extremities.

2. Functional assay for thiamine estimation is:

a. Serum thiamine
b. RBC transketolase level
c. RBC glutathione reductase
d. RNA editing

Ans. **b. RBC transketolase level**

Thiamine (Vitamin B1)

- Thiamine pyrophosphate (TPP) is the biologically active form of vitamin B1, formed by transfer of pyrophosphate group from ATP.

Functions of Thiamine

Thiamine diphosphate is the coenzyme for the following enzymes:
- Branched-chain ketoacid dehydrogenase involved in the metabolism of leucine, isoleucine and valine
- Alpha-ketoglutarate dehydrogenase in the citric acid cycle
- Pyruvate dehydrogenase in carbohydrate metabolism
- Transketolase reaction in the pentose phosphate pathway

Thiamine triphosphate has a role in nerve conduction—it phosphorylates and activates a chloride channel in the nerve membrane.

Thiamine nutritional status is best assessed by erythrocyte or whole blood transketolase activity.

Thiamine Deficiency Diseases

Beriberi:
- *Wet beriberi*: High-output congestive heart failure, peripheral edema and peripheral neuritis.
- *Dry beriberi*: Symmetric peripheral neuropathy of the motor and sensory systems, with diminished reflexes. Neuropathy mainly affects the lower limbs.
- *Infantile beriberi*: Occurs in infants born to mothers who are thiamine deficient. Features include tachycardia, vomiting, convulsions and death.

Wernicke encephalopathy with Korsakoff's psychosis:
- Alcoholic patients with chronic thiamine deficiency also may have CNS manifestations known as Wernicke's encephalopathy.
- *Wernicke's encephalopathy*: Involves periaqueductal gray matter, and presents with horizontal nystagmus, ophthalmoplegia (due to weakness of one or more extraocular muscles), cerebellar ataxia, and mental impairment.
- It then progreses into Korsakoff psychosis consisting of loss of memory and confabulations, a syndrome is known as Wernicke-Korsakoff syndrome.

3. Hepcidin decreases iron absorption by inhibition of:

a. Hephaestin
b. Ferroportin
c. Divalent metal ion transporter
d. Transferrin

Ans. b. Ferroportin

Iron Absorption

Iron absorption from the intestine is summarized in the following diagram:

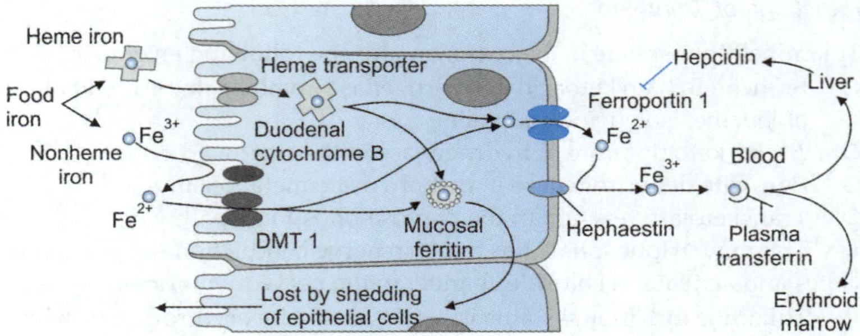

Regulation of Iron Absorption

- Hepcidin, synthesized by the liver, is the major regulator of iron absorption. Its levels are regulated by intrahepatic iron levels.
- Hepcidin binds to ferroportin, resulting in its endocytosis, thus inhibiting iron transfer from enterocyte to plasma. Iron becomes trapped within duodenal cells and is subsequently lost as these cells are sloughed.
- Conversely, with low body stores of iron, hepcidin synthesis falls and this in turn facilitates iron absorption.
- Hepcidin also acts on macrophages, suppressing iron release. It thus reduces the amount of iron available for erythroid precursors for hemoglobin synthesis.
- In iron deficiency, there is upregulation of Transferrin mRNA and receptor expression. Thus, transferrin receptor maintains cellular iron homeostasis.
- While ferritin synthesis decreases as it is a storage form of Iron. There is no change in ferritin mRNA concentration.
- TfR production in the cell is regulated according to iron levels by iron- responsive element-binding proteins, IRP1 and IRP2.

Ferroportin and Ceruloplasmin: Iron that enters the duodenal cells can follow one of two pathways: transport to the blood or storage as mucosal iron. This distribution is influenced by body iron stores. Fe^{2+} iron destined for the circulation is transported from the cytoplasm across the basolateral enterocyte membrane by **ferroportin**. This process is coupled to the oxidation of Fe^{2+} iron to Fe^{3+} iron, which is carried out by the iron oxidases hephaestin and **ceruloplasmin**.

4. Which of the following TCA cycle intermediate is a part of heme metabolism?

a. Succinyl CoA
b. Fumarate
c. Alpha ketoglutarate
d. Malate

Ans. a. Succinyl CoA

Heme Biosynthesis

- Heme biosynthesis occurs in most mammalian cells except RBCs, which do not contain mitochondria.
- *Sites*: 85% of heme synthesis occurs in erythroid precursor cells in the bone marrow, and the majority of the remainder in hepatocytes.
- The enzymatic process that produces heme is properly called porphyrin synthesis. In humans, this pathway serves almost exclusively to form heme.
- The pathway is initiated by the synthesis of δ-Aminolevulinic acid (δALA) from glycine and succinyl- CoA.
- This step is catalyzed by the rate-limiting enzyme of the pathway, ALA synthase, which is negatively regulated by glucose and heme concentration.
- It takes place in both cytoplasm and mitochondria.
- Most important heme containing molecule is hemoglobin, but it also forms part of other biologically important proteins such as myoglobin, cytochrome, catalase and endothelial nitric oxide synthase.

Steps of heme synthesis are depicted in the following diagram:

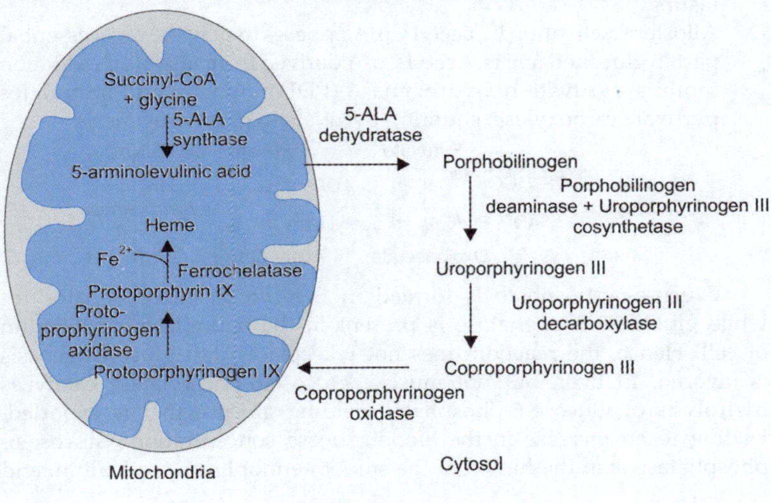

5. Enzyme involved in gluconeogenesis are all *except*:

a. Pyruvate carboxylase
b. PEP carboxykinase
c. Pyruvate kinase
d. Glucose-6 phosphatase

Ans. c. Pyruvate kinase

In gluconeogenesis, the steps of glycolysis are reversed to regenerate glucose from various molecules to supply energy for various tissues of the body. All steps in glycolysis are reversible except three, which are circumvented by reactions undertaken by the following molecules.

Regulatory and adaptive enzymes associated with gluconeogenesis				
	Inducer	***Repressor***	***Activator***	***Inhibitor***
Pyruvate carboxylase	Glucocorticoids, glucagon, epinephrine	Insulin	Acetyl CoA	ADP
Phosphoenol pyruvate carboxykinase	Glucocorticoids, glucagon, epinephrine	Insulin	Glucagon	
Glucose 6-phosphatase	Glucocorticoids, glucagon, epinephrine	Insulin		

- Liver and kidneys are the major gluconeogenic tissues.
- Glucogenic key enzymes are expressed in small intestine but their role in fasting state is unclear.
- Gluconeogenesis prevent hypoglycemia during short and long-term fasting.
- Allosteric activation by acetyl Co-A appears to play the most essential part in gluconeogensis: Acetyl Co-A derived from fatty acid oxidation inhibits pyruvate dehydrogenase (PDH) enzyme and stimulates pyruvate carboxylase, shunting pyruvate to gluconeogenesis.

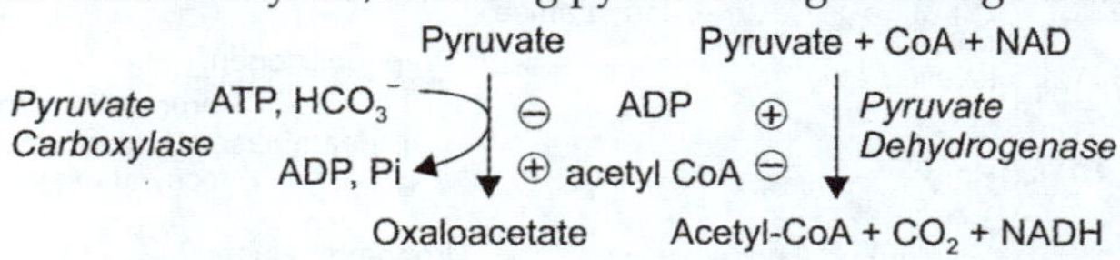

Glucose-6-phosphate is formed in the cytoplasm of hepatocytes while glucose-6-phosphatase is present in the endoplasmic reticulum of cell. Hence, the reaction does not take place until gluconeogenesis is favored. In liver, but not muscle, glucose-6-phosphatase catalyzes hydrolysis of glucose-6-phosphate, yielding glucose that is exported, leading to an increase in the blood glucose concentration. Glucose-6-phosphatase is in the lumen of the smooth endoplasmic reticulum, and genetic defects of the glucose-6-phosphate transporter can cause a variant of type I glycogen storage disease.

Substrates of gluconeogenesis

- Glucogenic amino acids (all except leucine and lysine which are purely ketogenic); most important is alanine
- Lactate
- Pyruvate
- Propionate
- Glycerol
- Fumarate

6. Exclusive mother to children's transmission is a key feature of which pattern of inheritance?

a. Codominance
b. Autosomal dominant inheritance
c. Recessive inheritance
d. Mitochondrial inheritance

Ans. d. Mitochondrial inheritance

Human Mitochondrial DNA

- It is circular, double-stranded.
- Contains 16 kbp (nuclear genome- 3.3 billion bp)
- Encodes 13 protein subunits of the respiratory chain (of a total of about 67 i.e. 20%)
- Encodes large (16S) and small (12S) mt ribosomal RNAs
- Encodes 22 mt tRNA molecules
- Genetic code differs slightly from the standard code
  - UGA (standard stop codon) is read as Trp
  - AGA and AGG (standard codons for Arg) are read as stop codons
- Contains very few untranslated sequences (3% noncoding vs 93% in nuclear DNA)
- High mutation rate (5–10 times that of nuclear DNA)
- Inheritance is strictly maternal—During fertilization, cytoplasm of the embryo is formed entirely by that of the ovum. Hence, only the maternal mitochondria is inherited by the embryo.

7. Which of the following hormones is secreted by the female adrenal gland?

a. Progesterone
b. Testosterone
c. Estrogen
d. DHEA

Ans. d. DHEA

Adrenal Steroidogenesis

- Cholesterol is mostly derived from plasma, but a small portion is synthesized in situ from acetyl-CoA via mevalonate and squalene.
- Much of cholesterol in adrenal is esterified and stored in cytoplasmic lipid droplets
  - Upon stimulation of adrenal by ACTH, an esterase is activated and free cholesterol formed is transported into mitochondrion, where a cytochrome P450 side chain cleavage enzyme (P4SOscc) converts cholesterol to pregnenolone.
- Cleavage of the side chain involves sequential hydroxylations first at C22 and then at C20, followed by side chain cleavage (removal of the six-carbon fragment iso caproaldehyde) to give 21-carbon steroid.
- An ACTH-dependent steroidogenic acute regulatory (StAR) protein is essential for transport of cholesterol to P450scc in inner mitochondrial membrane.
  - All mammalian steroid hormones are formed from cholesterol via pregnenolone through a series of reactions that occur in either mitochondria or endoplasmic reticulum of adrenal cell as depicted below:

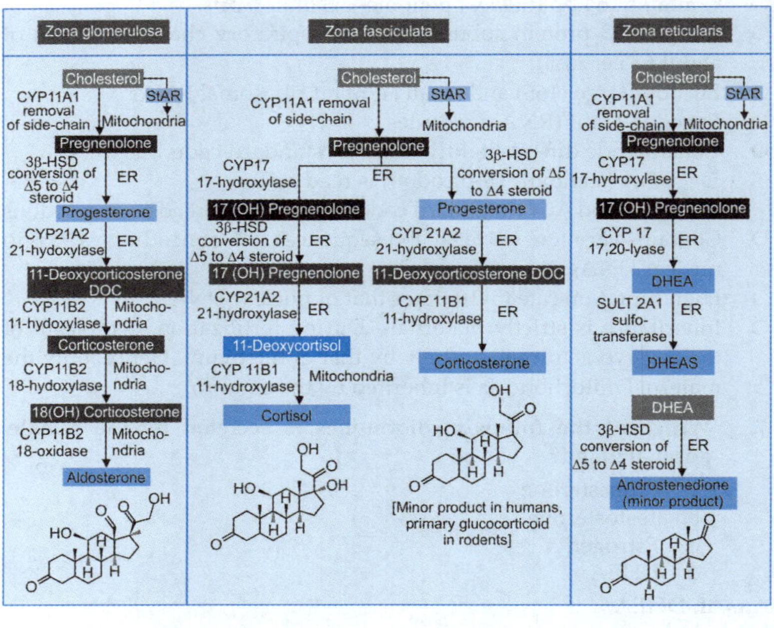

8. The graph shown below is the titration curve of glycine. Which of the following statements are true?

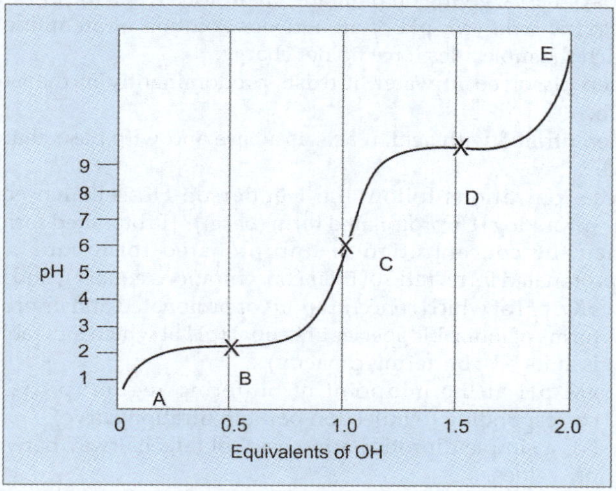

a. Point A represents the region where glycine is deprotonated
b. Points C represent the region of maximum buffer activity
c. Point C represents the region where the net charge on glycine is zero
d. Point D represents the pK of glycine's carboxyl group
e. Point E represents the pI for glycine.

Ans. a-F, b-T, c-T, d-F, e-F

- C represents the isoelectric point or pI, and as such is midway between pk1 and pk2 for glycine
- Glycine is fully protonated at Point A. Point C represents a region of maximum buffering.
- Point E represents the region where glycine is fully deprotonated

Titration Curve of Amino Acids

- Titration curves are obtained when the pH of a given volume of a sample solution varies on addition of acid or alkali.
- pH is plotted against the volume of the titrant added or the number of equivalents added per mole of the sample.
- *The shape of the curve depends upon*: Number of ionizing groups, pKa of ionizing group and buffer region.
- *Amino acids are weak polyprotic acids*: At neutral pH, they exist as zwitterions with equal number of negative and positive charges. They are amphoteric in character and can be titrated with both acid and alkali.

- All amino acids have an acidic group (COOH) and a basic group (NH_2) attached to a carbon and contain ionizable groups that act as weak acids or bases, giving off or taking on protons when the pH is altered.
- *Isoelectric point (pl)*: pH of an aqueous solution of an amino acid at which the molecules have no net charge.
- When dissolved in water, it exists predominantly in the isoelectric form.
- When titrated with acid, it acts as a base and with base, it acts as an acid.
- These ionizations follow the Henderson-Hesselbalch equation: pH = pKa + log [Unprotonated form (base)] / [Protonated form (acid)]
- When the concentration of unprotonated form equals that of unprotonated form, ratio of their concentrations equals 1, and log 1 = 0.
  - *pKa*: pH at which concentrations of protonated and unprotonated forms of ionizable species are equal (pH at which ionizable group is at its best buffering capacity)
  - *pK*: pH at the midpoint of buffering region (pK is the pH corresponding to inflection point in titration curve)
  - For a simple diprotic amino acid, pl falls halfway between two pK values.

A theoretical titration curve for glycine is given below:

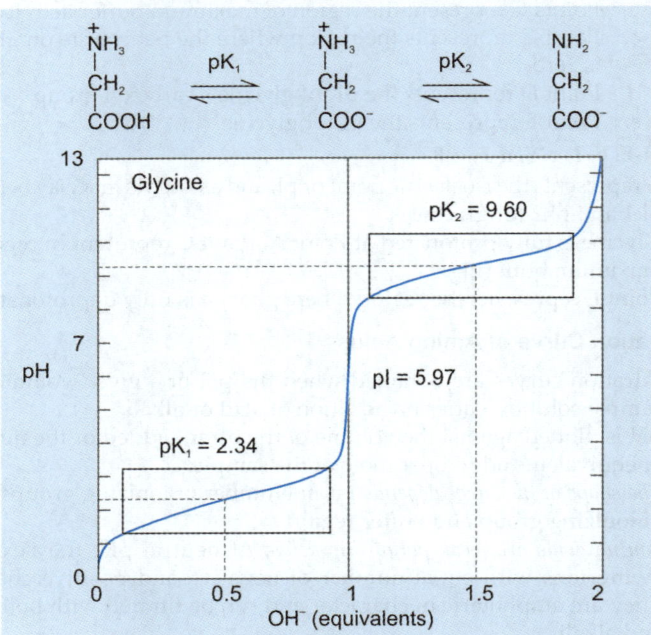

9. Kcat/km is a measure of:

a. Enzyme efficiency
b. Speed of enzymatic reaction
c. Concentration of substrate
d. Enzyme turn over

Ans. **a. Enzyme efficiency**

The Michaelis-Menten Equation

The Michaelis-Menten equation illustrates in mathematical terms the relationship between initial reaction velocity v_i and substrate concentration [S]:

$$v_i = \frac{V_{max}[S]}{K_m + [S]}$$

The Michaelis constant K_m is the substrate concentration at which v_i is half the maximal velocity ($V_{max}/2$) attainable at a particular concentration of the enzyme. K_m thus has the dimensions of substrate concentration.

Effect of substrate concentration on the initial velocity of an enzyme-catalyzed reaction:

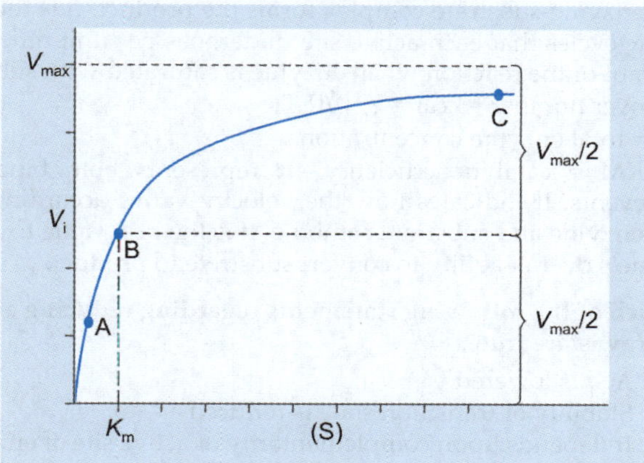

The dependence of initial reaction velocity on [S] and K_m may be illustrated by evaluating the Michaelis-Menten equation under three conditions:

1. When [S] is much less than K_m (point A in Figure), the term K_m + [S] is essentially equal to K_m. Replacing K_m + [S] with K_m reduces equation to

$$v_i = \frac{V_{max}[S]}{K_m + [S]} \quad v_i \approx \frac{V_{max}[S]}{K_m} \approx \left[\frac{V_{max}}{K_m}\right][S]$$

where ≈ means "approximately equal to." Since V_{max} and K_m are both constants, their ratio is a constant. In other words, when [S] is considerably below K_m, v_i is proportionate to k[S]. The initial reaction velocity therefore is directly proportional to [S].

2. When [S] is much greater than K_m (point C in Figure), the term K_m + [S] is essentially equal to [S]. Replacing K_m + [S] with [S] reduces equation to

$$v_i = \frac{F_{max}[S]}{K_m + [S]} \quad v_i \approx \frac{V_{max}[S]}{[S]} \approx V_{max}$$

Thus, when [S] greatly exceeds K_m, the reaction velocity is maximal (V_{max}) and unaffected by further increases in the substrate concentration.

3. When [S] = K_m (point B in Figure):

$$v_i = \frac{F_{max}[S]}{K_m + [S]} = \frac{V_{max}[S]}{[S]} \approx \frac{V_{max}}{2}$$

When [S] equals K_m, the initial velocity is half-maximal. Equation also reveals that K_m is—and may be determined experimentally from—the substrate concentration at which the initial velocity is half-maximal.

Turnover number/ catalytic constant (kcat) – It represents the speed in which enzyme-substrate complex forms the product. It is the number of catalytic cycles that each active site undergoes per unit time. It is the rate constant of the reaction when enzyme is saturated with substrate.

Turnover number = kcat = V_{max}/[ET]

[ET] = total enzyme concentration

kcat/KM = catalytic efficiency—It represents both binding and catalytic events. It indicates how the velocity varies according to how often the enzyme and substrate combine. It is the best value to represent the enzyme's overall ability to convert substrate to product.

10. Which of the following statements regarding reducing activation energy is/are true?

a. ΔG_F is lowered
b. Stability of transition state is reduced
c. It depends upon complementarity of active site of enzyme and substrate
d. Conformational change may occur at the active site of enzyme at the time of binding to substrate

Ans. **a-T, b-F, c-T, d-T**

Enzyme Catalysis

Reactions proceed via formation of an intermediate molecule. This transient intermediate—in which neither free substrate nor product exists—is termed the transition state. ΔG refers to the change in free energy when substrate is converted into product. ΔG_F refers to difference between the free energy of substrate and transition state. Regardless of the sign or magnitude of ΔG, ΔG_F for the overwhelming majority of chemical reactions has a positive sign, which indicates that formation of the transition state requires surmounting one or more energy barriers. For this reason, ΔG_F for reaching a transition state is often termed the activation energy, E_{act}. The ease—and hence the frequency—with which this barrier is overcome is inversely related to E_{act}. For a simple reaction,

$$\text{Rate} \propto e^{-E_{act}/RT}$$

The activation energy for the reaction proceeding in the opposite direction to that drawn is equal to $-\Delta G_D$. Enzymes Lower the Activation Energy Barrier for a Reaction. All enzymes accelerate reaction rates by lowering ΔG_F for the formation of transition states. However, they may differ in the way this is achieved. While the sequence of chemical steps at the active site parallels those which occur when the substrates react in the absence of a catalyst, the environment of the active site lowers ΔG_F by stabilizing the transition state intermediates. The enzyme binds to the transition state intermediate more tightly than it does to either substrates or products. Catalysis by enzymes that proceeds via a unique reaction mechanism typically occurs when the transition state intermediate forms a covalent bond with the enzyme (covalent catalysis).

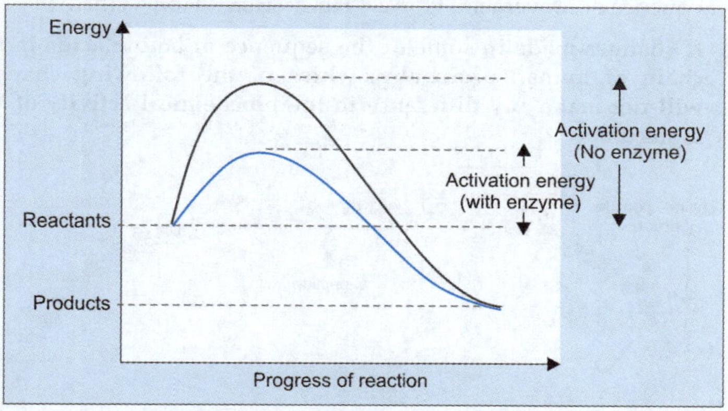

11. Which type of mutation occurs in sickle cell anemia?

a. Insertion
b. Deletion
c. Point mutation
d. Frame shift

Ans. c. Point mutation

Sickle Cell Anemia

- Characterized by point mutation in the beta globin chain of hemoglobin, which results in coding of valine instead of glutamate at position 6.

- Autosomal recessive inheritance.
- This replacement creates a 'Sticky hydrophobic patch' (contact point) on the outer surface at position 6 of β-chain of both oxy HbS and deoxy HbS (but not in Hb A).
- Complementary sticky patch is found in both HbA and HbS, but is exposed only in their deoxygenated (T) state.
- HbA remains a true solute at rather higher concentrations because of polar exterior surface that is compatible and nonreactive with nearby Hb molecules. In contrast HbS when deoxygenated is less soluble.
- Thus, at low PO_2, deoxy HbS can polymerize to form long, insoluble fibers. These twisted helical fibers distort the erythrocyte into characteristic sickle shape.
- The mobility of HbS as compared with normal hemoglobin on gel electrophoresis will be decreased. During electrophoresis at alkaline pH, Hb S migrates more slowly toward the anode (positive electrode) than does HbA. This altered mobility of Hb S is a result of the absence of the negatively charged glutamate residues in the two β chains, thus rendering Hb S less negative than Hb A.
- Sequence of Movement: HbA2 < HbC < HbS < HbF < HbA.

12. If changes made in some of the sequence of amino acids in the chain of human proinsulin, which of the following changes will not make any difference in the biochemical activity of the molecule?

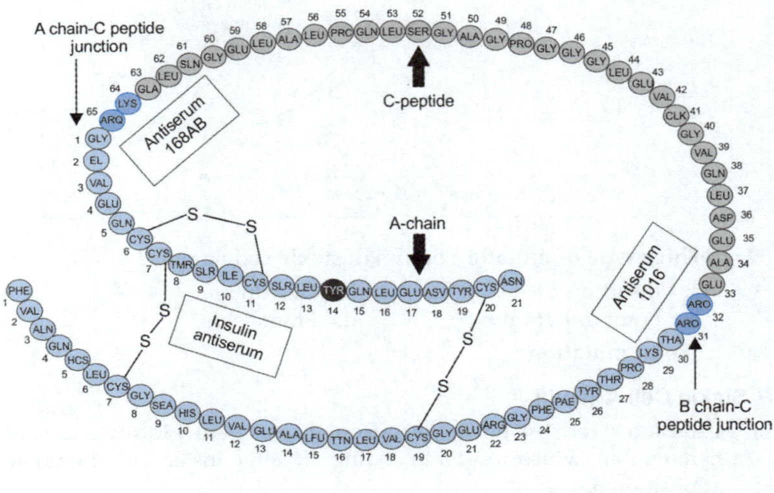

a. Breaking disulfide linkage
b. Interchange of A1 and A4
c. Interchange of B29 and B30
d. Interchange of A5 and A6

Ans. c. Interchange of B29 and B30

Insulin has an AB heterodimeric structure with one intrachain (A6-A11) and two interchain disulfide bridges (A7-B7 and A20-B19). Insulin is synthesized as a preprohormone, which is the prototype for peptides that are processed from larger precursor molecules. The hydrophobic 23-amino-acid pre-, or leader, sequence directs the molecule into the cisternae of the endoplasmic reticulum and then is removed. This results in the 9000-MW proinsulin molecule, which provides the conformation necessary for the proper and efficient formation of the disulfide bridges. The sequence of proinsulin, starting from the amino terminus, is B chain—connecting (C) peptide—A chain. The proinsulin molecule undergoes a series of site-specific peptide cleavages that result in the formation of equimolar amounts of mature insulin and C-peptide. Insulin and C-peptide molecules are connected at two sites by peptide bonds. An initial cleavage by a trypsin-like enzyme followed by several cleavages by a carboxypeptidase-like enzyme results in the production of the heterodimeric (AB) insulin molecule, which is held together by two intrapeptide cysteine disulfide bonds; insulin C-peptide.

Regarding the options, breaking disulfide bonds will affect the shape and stability of the molecule, hence the function. Therefore, options a and d will cause changes. A1 to A4: the A chain provides the more extensive receptor-binding surface. The key A-chain recognition element comprises A1-A4. The segment B26–B30 can be successfully removed without affecting the function of the insulin.

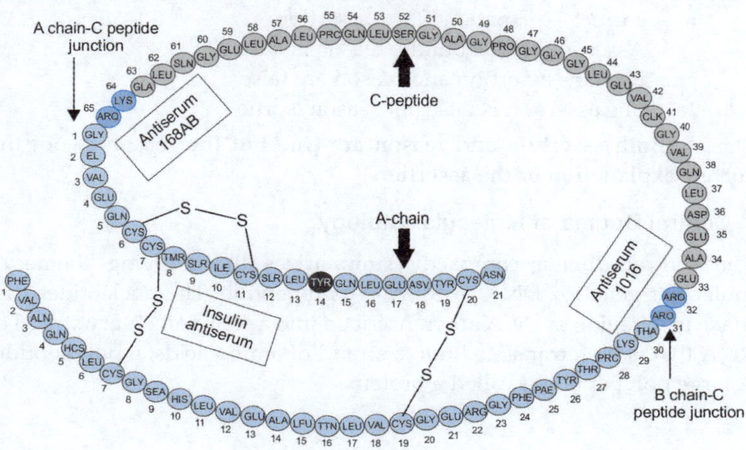

13. Which of the following processes does not happen from 5′ to 3′ direction?

a. DNA replication
b. DNA repair
c. RNA editing
d. Transcription

Ans. c. RNA editing

- In RNA editing, the editosome can edit only in 3′→ 5′ direction, along with primary RNA transcript.
- DNA replication goes in the 5′ to 3′ direction because DNA polymerase acts on the 3′-OH of the existing strand for adding free nucleotides.
- In transcription the complementary RNA is created in the opposite direction, in the 5′ → 3′ direction, matching the sequence of the sense strand with the exception of switching uracil for thymine.
- Mismatch DNA repair also occurs in 5′ → 3′ direction. When the strand containing the mismatch is identified, an endonuclease nicks the strand and the mismatched nucleotide(s) is/are removed by an exonuclease.

14. Assertion: According to central dogma, information flows from DNA to RNA, which is then encoded into protein.
Reason: In retrovirus, reverse of central dogma happens:

a. Both the assertion and the reason are true and the reason is a correct explanation of the assertion
b. Both assertion and reason are true but the reason is not the correct explanation of the assertion
c. Assertion is true but the reason is false
d. Both the assertion and reason are false
e. The assertion is false but reason is true

Ans. b. Both assertion and reason are true but the reason is not the correct explanation of the assertion

Central Dogma of Molecular Biology

The central dogma compactly summarizes the unifying theme of molecular genetics: DNA ↔ RNA → polypeptide. The nucleotides that make up a region of DNA are transcribed into a complementary strand of RNA that is then translated into a strand of amino acids, a polypeptide. A large polypeptide is called a protein.

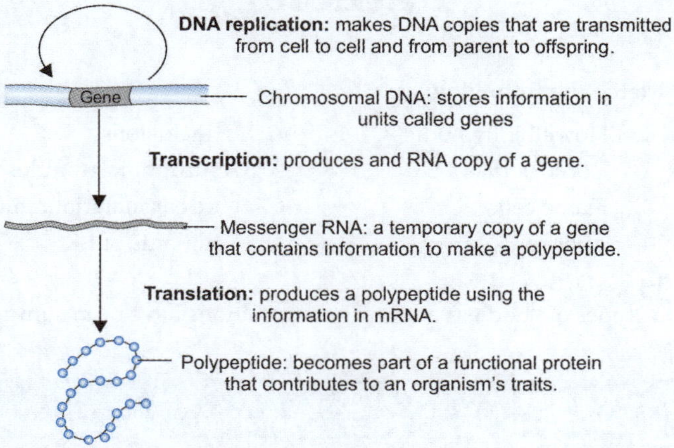

One portion of this information flow is reversible in special circumstances. Retroviruses that utilize RNA as their genetic material use reverse transcriptase to create a DNA copy that can integrate into the host's genome so it is transmitted to daughter cells during cell division. The other step, translation of the RNA sequence into protein, is not reversible.

Pathology

1. Match the following:

1.	Howell Jolly bodies	A.	Ig inclusions
2.	Dohle bodies	B.	Azurophilic granules
3.	Flame cells	C.	Nuclear material remnants
4.	Auer rods	D.	Remnants of ER

Ans. **1-C, 2-D, 3-A, 4-B**

Various types of "bodies" and their compositions have been summarized below:

Name of inclusion/ cell	Location	Composition	Associated disease
Auer rods	Myeloid blast cells	Azurophilic granules	AML
Flame cells, Mott cells	Plasma cell	Ig inclusions	Multiple myeloma
Dohle bodies	Neutrophils	ER remnants	Reactive leukocytosis
Howell-Jolly body	RBC	DNA	Hyposplenism/ asplenism
Heinz body	RBC	Denatured hemoglobin	G6PD deficiency
Basophilic stippling	RBC	RNA	Lead poisoning, thalassemia, sickle cell anemia
Pappenheimer body	RBC	Iron deposits	Thalassemia, sideroblastic anemia, hemolytic anemia
HbH body	RBC	Globin tetramers	Alpha thalassemia
Cabot rings	RBC	Mitotic spindle remnants	Megaloblastic anemia, myelodysplastic syndromes

2. A 40 years old gentleman came to the OPD with complains of itching during baths. His blood counts were-Hb: 20 g%, Platelets: 80,000/mm^3, WBC: 30,000/mm^3. Genetic analysis revealed Jak-2 mutation. What is the most likely diagnosis?

a. Essential thrombocytosis
b. Chronic myeloid leukemia
c. Polycythemia vera
d. Primary myelofibrosis

Ans. **c. Polycythemia vera**

Laboratory Features of Myeloproliferative Neoplasms

	WBC count	Hematocrit	Platelet count	Red cell morphology
Polycythemia vera	Normal/raised	Very high	Normal/ raised	Normal
Essential thrombocytosis	Normal/raised	Normal	Very high	Normal
Primary myelofibrosis	Normal/raised/ reduced	Reduced	Normal/raised/ reduced	Abnormal
Chronic myeloid leukemia	Very high	Normal/ reduced	Normal/raised/ reduced	Normal

Aquagenic pruritis is a specific diagnostic feature of polycythemia vera.

3. Acute inflammation seen in:

a. Necrosis
b. Apoptosis
c. Pyroptosis
d. Necroptosis

Ans. **a. Necrosis**

Irreversible Cell Death

Feature	Necrosis	Apoptosis
Cell size	Enlarged (swelling)	Reduced (shrinkage)
Nucleus	Pyknosis → karyorrhexis → karyolysis	Fragmentation into nucleosome-size fragments
Plasma membrane	Disrupted	Intact; altered structure, especially orientation of lipids
Cellular contents	Enzymatic digestion; may leak out of cell	Intact; may be released in apoptotic bodies
Adjacent inflammation	Frequent	No
Physiologic or pathologic role	Invariably pathologic (culmination of irreversible cell injury)	Often physiologic, means of eliminating unwanted cells; may be pathologic after some forms of cell injury, especially DNA damage
Agarose gel electro-phoresis of DNA	Diffuse smearing of DNA	Ladder pattern of DNA fragments

4. All of the following are seen in reversible injury *except*:

a. Loss of microvilli
b. Myelin figures
c. Plasma membrane blebs
d. Cell swelling

Ans. **b. Myelin figures**

Features of Reversible Cell Injury

Cellular swelling is the first manifestation of almost all forms of injury to cells. On microscopic examination, small clear vacuoles may be seen within the cytoplasm; these represent distended and pinched-off segments of the ER. This pattern of nonlethal injury is sometimes called hydropic change or vacuolar degeneration. Swelling of cells is reversible. Cells may also show increased eosinophilic staining, which becomes much more pronounced with progression to necrosis.

The ultrastructural changes of reversible cell injury include:

1. Plasma membrane alterations, such as blebbing, blunting, and loss of microvilli
2. Mitochondrial changes, including swelling and the appearance of small amorphous densities
3. Dilation of the ER, with detachment of polysomes; intracytoplasmic myelin figures may be present
4. Nuclear alterations, with disaggregation of granular and fibrillar elements.

5. Match the following types of endothelial dysfunction with their causes:

1. Sunburn	A. Immediate sustained
2. Bee sting	B. Delayed prolonged
3. Bacterial enzymes	C. Endothelial cell retraction
4. Tumor necrosis factor	D. Immediate transient

Ans. **1-B, 2-D, 3-A, 4-C**

Mechanisms of increased vascular permeability: Several mechanisms increase vascular permeability, some of which are physiologic and some of which are pathologic. Endothelial contraction and retraction are physiologic mechanisms and are due to mediators. Direct endothelial injury is a pathologic mechanism due to damaging agents not under the body's control.

- **Endothelial contraction** (referred to as immediate-transient response)
  - *Mediators*: Histamine, bradykinin, and leukotrienes.
  - *Vessels affected*: Postcapillary venules.
  - *Time course*: Immediate; short lived (up to 30 minutes).
- **Endothelial cell retraction**
  - *Mediators*: Tumor necrosis factor (TNF) and interleukins (e.g., IL-1).
  - *Mechanism*: Structural rearrangement of cytoskeleton.
  - *Time course*: 4–6 hours (referred to as delayed response); long lived.

- **Direct endothelial injury**
  - *Mediators*: Bacterial enzymes.
  - *Vessels affected*: All.
  - *Mechanism*: Endothelial cell necrosis.
  - *Time course*: Immediate (referred to as immediate-sustained response).
- **Delayed prolonged response**
  - Due to ultraviolet light, X-ray, and mild thermal injury.
  - Uncertain mechanism.
- **Leukocyte-mediated damage**

6. What is the use of the marked component in the blood transfusion set?

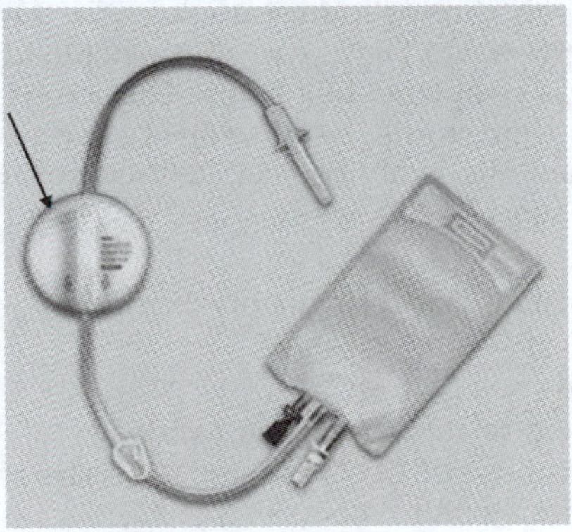

a. Decrease inflammation
b. Decrease the risk of viral infection
c. Decrease the number of leucocytes
d. Prevent hemolysis

Ans. c. Decrease the number of leucocytes

Leukocyte reduction of blood components is widely practiced to achieve a number of benefits. These include prevention of febrile reactions, avoiding leukocyte induced alloimmunization, reducing transmission of cytomegalovirus to levels comparable to those achieved through use of seronegative units. Immunosuppression induced by allogeneic transfusion may also be abrogated by leukoreduction. Since 1950s, it has been clearly established that removal of buffy coat from the whole blood, removes 70–80% of the WBCs and is sufficient in preventing many febrile non-hemolytic transfusion reactions (FNHTRs) to blood but not HLA alloimmunization or cytomegalovirus transmission.

Filtration has emerged as the most commonly used method of leukocyte reduction. Leukocyte reduction by means of filtration can be performed at three different points in time—before storage, after storage but before issue for the blood bank, and at the bedside. Prestorage leukofiltration may offer additional benefits over leukocyte removal during or after the storage period in terms of avoiding the potential of reaction and alloimmunization, in several ways. Firstly, HLA antigens may solubilize from leukocyte membranes during storage, passing through a filter applied after storage and immunizing the recipient. Secondly, cytokines released from leukocytes during storage, may cause FNHTR in transfusion recipients. Furthermore, release of enzymes by the leukocytes during storage may be detrimental to red cell metabolism and viability. In addition, conducting the filtration in laboratory rather than at bedside, permits quality control checks and tighter control over the performance of the technique and leads to more uniform results.

7. A patient with chronic kidney disease was posted for dialysis. Since his Hb was 5.2 g%, two units of blood were arranged. First bag was completed in 2 hours. The second bag was started and after a short while, he developed shortness of breath and hypertension. His vitals are—BP 180/100 mm Hg, PR 110/min. What is the most likely cause?

a. TRALI
b. Transfusion-related circulatory overload
c. Allergic reaction
d. FNHTR

Ans. b. Transfusion-related circulatory overload

The criteria for diagnosis of TACO states that it is characterized by any of the 4 of the following within 6 hours of transfusion:

1. Acute respiratory distress
2. Tachycardia
3. Raised blood pressure
4. Acute or worsening pulmonary edema on CXR
5. Evidence of positive fluid balance

This is usually due to rapid or massive transfusion of blood in patients with diminished cardiac reserve or chronic anemia. Patients over 60 years of age, infants and severely anemic patients are particularly susceptible.

8. True/false about amyloidosis:

a. β_2 macroglobulin forms amyloid in systemic senile amyloidosis
b. In AL type, amyloid is most commonly formed from kappa chain
c. Apple green birefringence is seen when Congo Red stain is used
d. SAA forms amyloid in multiple myeloma
e. Most common cause of amyloidosis is secondary

Ans. a-F, b-F, c-T, d-F, e-F

Amyloidosis

Approximately 95% of the amyloid material consists of fibril proteins, the remaining 5% being the P component and other glycoproteins. Three most common types are: (1) AL (amyloid light chain) is derived from Ig light chains produced in plasma cells; (2) AA (amyloid-associated) is derived from a unique non-Ig protein synthesized by the liver; and (3) Aβ amyloid is produced from β amyloid precursor protein and is found in the cerebral lesions of Alzheimer disease.

- The AL protein is made up of complete immunoglobulin light chains, the amino-terminal fragments of light chains, or both. Most of the AL proteins analyzed are composed of λ light chains or their fragments, but in some cases κ chains have been identified. The amyloid fibril protein of the AL type is produced from free Ig light chains secreted by a monoclonal population of plasma cells, and its deposition is associated with certain forms of plasma cell tumors.
- The second major class of amyloid fibril protein (AA) does not have structural homology to immunoglobulins. AA fibrils are derived by proteolysis from a larger precursor in the serum called SAA (serum amyloid–associated) protein that is synthesized in the liver and circulates in association with high density lipoproteins. The production of SAA protein is increased in inflammatory states as part of the "acute phase response"; therefore, this form of amyloidosis is associated with chronic inflammation, and is often called secondary amyloidosis.
- β-amyloid protein (Aβ) constitutes the core of cerebral plaques found in Alzheimer disease as well as the amyloid deposited in walls of cerebral blood vessels in individuals with this disease. The Aβ protein is derived by proteolysis from a much larger transmembrane glycoprotein, called amyloid precursor protein.
- Transthyretin (TTR) is a normal serum protein that binds and transports thyroxine and retinol. A mutant form of TTR (and its fragments) is deposited in a group of genetically determined disorders referred to as familial amyloid polyneuropathies. TTR is also deposited in the heart of aged individuals (senile systemic amyloidosis), but in such cases the amino acid sequence of the TTR molecule is normal.
- β_2-microglobulin, a component of MHC class I molecules and a normal serum protein, has been identified as the amyloid fibril subunit ($A\beta_2m$) in amyloidosis that complicates the course of patients on long-term hemodialysis.

9. Which of the following are the cell markers of T Regulatory cell?

a. CD4, CD25 b. FOX2, IL-2
c. CD8 d. CD4

Ans. **a. CD4, CD25**

Markers for Various Blood Cells

Types of cell	CD markers
Stem cells	CD34+, CD31–, CD17
All leukocyte groups	CD45+ (LCA)
Granulocyte	CD45+, CD11b, CD15+, CD24+, CD114+, CD182+
Monocyte	CD4, CD45+, CD14+, CD114+, CD11a, CD11b, CD91+, CD16+
T lymphocyte	CD45+, CD3+ (Pan-T-cell); CD1, 2, 3, 4, 5, 7, 8
T helper cell	CD45 +, CD3+, CD4+ ,
T regulatory cell	CD4, CD25, FOXP3
Cytotoxic T-cell	CD45+, CD3+, CD8+
Memory T-cell	CD45RO
B lymphocyte	CD45+, CD19+, CD2O+, CD24+, CD38 CD21, CD22, CD10 (Early B-cell)
Thrombocyte	CD45+, CD61+
Natural killer cell	CD1+, CD56+, CD3–, CD31, CD30, CD38
Langerhans cell histiocytosis	CD1a, S100, CD207 (Langerin)
Reed Sternberg cells	CD15, CD30

10. Which of the following antibodies is involved in allergic hypersensitivity?

a. IgM
b. IgA
c. IgG
d. IgE

Ans. d. IgE

Hypersensitivity Reactions

Type	Mechanism	Clinical manifestation or disease
I (Allergic, anaphylactic)	Antigen (allergen) induces IgE antibody that binds to mast cells and basophils. When exposed to the allergen again, the allergen cross-links the bound IgE on those cells. This causes degranulation and release of mediators (e.g., histamine)	Systemic anaphylaxis, urticaria (hives), asthma, hay fever, allergic rhinitis, allergic conjunctivitis, food allergies (e.g., nuts, shellfish, eggs), drug allergies especially penicillin, eczema (atopic dermatitis), bee venom, latex gloves, angioedema
II (Cytotoxic)	Antigens on a cell surface combine with IgG antibody. This leads to complement-mediated lysis of the cells	Hemolytic anemia, neutropenia, thrombocytopenia, ABO transfusion reactions, Rh incompatibility (erythroblastosis fetalis, hemolytic disease of the newborn), rheumatic fever, Goodpasture's syndrome

Contd...

Contd...

Type	Mechanism	Clinical manifestation or disease
III (Immune complex)	Antigen–antibody immune complexes are deposited in tissues, complement is activated, and polymorphonuclear cells are attracted to the site. They release lysosomal enzymes, causing tissue damage	Systemic lupus erythematosus, rheumatoid arthritis, poststreptococcal glomerulonephritis, IgA nephropathy, serum sickness, hypersensitivity pneumonitis (e.g., farmer's lung), Arthus reaction
IV (Delayed)	T lymphocytes activated/ sensitized by an antigen release lymphokines upon second contact with the same antigen. The lymphokines induce inflammation and activate macrophages, which, in turn, release various inflammatory mediators	Contact dermatitis, poison oak/ ivy, tuberculin skin test reaction, drug rash, Stevens-Johnson syndrome, toxic epidermal necrolysis, erythema multiforme

11. Chimerism is helpful in:

a. Solid organ transplant
b. Maternity testing
c. Personal identification
d. Paternity testing

Ans. a. Solid organ transplant

Donor Cell Chimerism

Immunosuppression after solid organ transplant has concomitant risks of opportunistic infections and secondary tumors. Therefore, the ultimate goal of research on organ transplantation and autoimmune diseases is to induce and maintain immunological tolerance, the active state of antigen-specific non-responsiveness. A promising approach is induction of chimerism (coexistence of cells from two genetic lineages in a single individual) by first dampening or eliminating immune function in the recipient with ionizing radiation, drugs such as cyclophosphamide, or antibody treatment and then providing a new source of immune function by adoptive transfer (transfusion) of bone marrow or hematopoietic stem cells. On reconstitution of immune function, the recipient no longer recognizes new antigens provided during a critical period as "non self." Such tolerance is long lived and less likely to be complicated by the use of calcineurin inhibitors.

12. Which of the following molecules is responsible for cell cycle arrest after DNA damage?

a. p53
b. p16
c. Rb
d. p64

Ans. a. p53

p53 Tumor Suppressor Gene

The p53 gene is located on chromosome 17p13.1, and it is the most common target for genetic alteration in human tumors. Over 50% of human tumors contain mutations in this gene. Homozygous loss of p53 occurs in virtually every type of cancer, including carcinomas of the lung, colon, and breast—the three leading causes of cancer death. p53 links cell damage with DNA repair, cell cycle arrest, and apoptosis. In response to DNA damage, p53 is phosphorylated by genes that sense the damage and are involved in DNA repair. p53 assists in DNA repair by causing G1 arrest and inducing DNA repair genes. A cell with damaged DNA that cannot be repaired is directed by p53 to undergo apoptosis. In view of these activities, p53 has been rightfully called a "guardian of the genome." With loss of function of p53, DNA damage goes unrepaired, mutations accumulate in dividing cells, and the cell marches along a one-way street leading to malignant transformation.

The ability of p53 to control apoptosis in response to DNA damage has important practical therapeutic implications. Irradiation and chemotherapy, the two common modalities of cancer treatment, mediate their effects by inducing DNA damage and subsequent apoptosis. Tumors that retain normal p53 are more likely to respond to such therapy than tumors that carry mutated alleles of the gene. Such is the case with testicular teratocarcinomas and childhood acute lymphoblastic leukemias. By contrast, tumors such as lung cancers and colorectal cancers, which frequently carry p53 mutations, are relatively resistant to chemotherapy and irradiation. Various therapeutic modalities aimed at increasing normal p53 activity in tumor cells that retain this type of activity or selectively killing cells with defective p53 function are being investigated.

13. Which of the following is the cause for development of berry aneurysm?

a. Mucoid degeneration of medial layer
b. Defect in adventitial layer
c. Internal elastic lamina defect
d. Intimal damage

Ans. **c. Internal elastic lamina defect**

Berry Aneurysm

Berry aneurysms are intracranial aneurysms, most commonly involving the circle of Willis. It has a prevalence of 2% in adults. Unruptured, asymptomatic aneurysms are much less dangerous than a recently ruptured aneurysm. Aneurysm location may also factor into risk, with basilar bifurcation aneurysms appearing to have a somewhat higher rupture risk. Because of the longer length of exposure to risk of rupture, younger patients with aneurysms >10 mm in size may benefit from prophylactic treatment. Giant aneurysms, those >2.5 cm in diameter, occur at the same sites (see below) as small aneurysms and account for 5% of cases. The three most common locations are the terminal internal carotid artery, middle cerebral artery (MCA) bifurcation, and top of the basilar artery. Their risk of rupture is ~6% in the first year after identification and may remain high indefinitely. They often cause symptoms by compressing the adjacent brain or cranial nerves.

Saccular aneurysms occur at the bifurcations of the large- to medium-sized intracranial arteries; rupture is into the subarachnoid space in the basal cisterns and sometimes into the parenchyma of the adjacent brain. Approximately 85% of aneurysms occur in the anterior circulation, mostly on the circle of Willis. About 20% of patients have multiple aneurysms, many at mirror sites bilaterally. As an aneurysm develops, it typically forms a neck with a dome. The length of the neck and the size of the dome vary greatly and are important factors in planning neurosurgical obliteration or endovascular embolization. The arterial internal elastic lamina disappears at the base of the neck. The media thins, and connective tissue replaces smooth-muscle cells. At the site of rupture (most often the dome), the wall thins, and the tear that allows bleeding is often ≤0.5 mm long. Aneurysm size and site are important in predicting risk of rupture. Those >7 mm in diameter and those at the top of the basilar artery and at the origin of the posterior communicating artery are at greater risk of rupture.

14. A 10-year-old child presents to the OPD with pedal edema and facial puffiness for the past 5 days. BP was 126/80 mm Hg. Proteinuria 3+. Urine examination shows 100 RBCs/hpf. What is the most likely diagnosis?

a. Poststreptococcal glomerulonephritis
b. Minimal change disease
c. Membranous glomerulonephritis
d. Focal segmental glomerulosclerosis

Ans. **a. Poststreptococcal glomerulonephritis**

Poststreptococcal Glomerulonephritis

It usually appears 1 to 4 weeks after a streptococcal infection of the pharynx or skin (impetigo). Poststreptococcal glomerulonephritis occurs most frequently in children 6 to 10 years of age, but adults of any age can also be affected.

Pathogenesis

Only certain strains of group A β-hemolytic streptococci are nephritogenic, more than 90% of cases being traced to types 12, 4, and 1, which can be identified by typing of M protein of the cell wall. Poststreptococcal glomerulonephritis is an immunologically mediated disease. Several *cationic antigens*, including a nephritis-associated streptococcal plasmin receptor (NAPlr), unique to nephritogenic strains of streptococci, can be found in affected glomeruli. Other evidence suggests that streptococcal pyogenic exotoxin B (SpeB) and its zymogen precursor (zSpeB), another protein that functions as a plasmin receptor, are the principal antigenic determinants in most cases of poststreptococcal glomerulonephritis.

Histology

The major finding is **enlarged, hypercellular glomeruli**. The hypercellularity is caused by (1) infiltration by leukocytes, both neutrophils and monocytes; (2) proliferation of endothelial and mesangial cells; and (3) in severe cases by crescent formation.

By **immunofluorescence microscopy**, there are granular deposits of IgG, IgM, and C3 in the mesangium and along the GBM. Although immune complex deposits are almost universally present, they are often focal and sparse. The characteristic **electron microscopic findings** are discrete, amorphous, electron-dense deposits on the epithelial side of the membrane, often having the appearance of "humps" representing the antigen-antibody complexes at the epithelial cell surface.

Clinical Features

Clinical presentation involves malaise, fever, nausea, oliguria, and hematuria (smoky or cola-colored urine) 1 to 2 weeks after recovery from a sore throat. The patients have red cell casts in the urine, mild proteinuria (usually less than 1 gm/day), periorbital edema, and mild to moderate hypertension. Important laboratory findings include elevations of antistreptococcal antibody titers and a decline in the serum concentration of C3 and other components of the complement cascade. More than 95% of affected children eventually recover totally with conservative therapy aimed at maintaining sodium and water balance.

15. Dystrophic calcification is seen in: *(Updated)*

a. Paget disease b. Sarcoidosis
c. Myositis ossificans d. Immobilization after fracture

Ans. c. Myositis ossificans

Dystrophic Calcification

Dystrophic calcification is seen any type of necrosis- coagulative, caseous, liquefactive type, and necrosis of fat. Calcification is frequently seen in atheromas of advanced atherosclerosis. It also commonly develops in aging or damaged heart valves, further hampering their function. The calcium salts appear macroscopically as fine, white granules or clumps, often felt as gritty deposits. Sometimes a tuberculous lymph node is virtually converted to stone.

Metastatic Calcification

Metastatic calcification occurs in normal tissues in the setting of hypercalcemia. Hypercalcemia also accentuates dystrophic calcification. The major causes are:

1. Increased secretion of parathyroid hormone (PTH) with subsequent bone resorption, as in hyperparathyroidism due to parathyroid tumors, and ectopic secretion of PTH-related protein by malignant tumors
2. Destruction of bone tissue—secondary to primary tumors of bone marrow (e.g., multiple myeloma, leukemia) or diffuse skeletal metastasis (e.g., breast cancer), accelerated bone turnover (e.g., Paget disease), or immobilization
3. Vitamin D-related disorders, including vitamin D intoxication, sarcoidosis (in which macrophages activate a vitamin D precursor), and idiopathic hypercalcemia of infancy (Williams syndrome), characterized by abnormal sensitivity to vitamin D
4. Renal failure—causes retention of phosphate, leading to secondary hyperparathyroidism.

16. Which of the following lab test is used to assess the intrinsic pathway of coagulation?

a. aPTT
b. PT
c. Bleeding time
d. Clotting time

Ans. a. aPTT

Coagulation Assays

Based on assays carried out in clinical laboratories, the coagulation cascade has traditionally been divided into the extrinsic and intrinsic pathways.

The prothrombin time (PT) assay assesses the function of the proteins in the **extrinsic** pathway (factors VII, X, V, II, and fibrinogen). In brief, **tissue factor**, phospholipids, and **calcium** are added to plasma and the time for a fibrin clot to form is recorded.

The partial thromboplastin time (PTT) assay screens the function of the proteins in the intrinsic pathway (factors XII, XI, IX, VIII, X, V, II, and fibrinogen). In this assay, clotting of plasma is initiated by addition of negative charged particles (e.g., ground glass) that activate factor XII (Hageman factor) together with phospholipids and calcium, and the time to fibrin clot formation is recorded.

Pharmacology

1. Aspirin and phenobarbitone are acidic drugs whereas diazepam is a basic drug. Mention the true/false statements about these drugs:

a. Aspirin is present in mainly non-ionized form in stomach, hence can be easily absorbed
b. Diazepam is mostly absorbed from intestine
c. Phenobarbitone can be absorbed from the stomach but most of the absorption occurs in small intestine due to its large surface area
d. No drug is absorbed in the large intestine due to its very low surface area
e. Diseases decreasing the transit time of drugs like diarrhea will increase the drug absorption in the small intestine

Ans. **a-T, b-T, c-T, d-F, e-F**

Oral Administration of Drugs

Oral ingestion is the most common method of drug administration. It is also the safest, most convenient, and most economical. Its disadvantages include limited absorption of some drugs because of their physical characteristics (e.g., low water solubility or poor membrane permeability), emesis as a result of irritation to the GI mucosa, destruction of some drugs by digestive enzymes or low gastric pH, irregularities in absorption or propulsion in the presence of food or other drugs, and the need for cooperation on the part of the patient. In addition, drugs in the GI tract may be metabolized by the enzymes of the intestinal microbiome, mucosa, or liver before they gain access to the general circulation.

Absorption from the GI tract is governed by factors such as surface area for absorption; blood flow to the site of absorption; the physical state of the drug (solution, suspension, or solid dosage form); its aqueous solubility; and the drug's concentration at the site of absorption. For drugs given in solid form, the rate of dissolution may limit their absorption. Because most drug absorption from the GI tract occurs by passive diffusion, absorption is favored when the drug is in the nonionized, more lipophilic form. Based on the pH-partition concept, one would predict that drugs that are weak acids would be better absorbed from the stomach (pH 1–2) than from the upper intestine (pH 3–6), and vice versa for weak bases. However, the surface area of the stomach is relatively small, and a mucus layer covers the gastric epithelium. By contrast, the villi of the upper intestine provide an extremely large surface area (~200 m^2). Accordingly, the rate of absorption of a drug from the intestine will be greater than that from the stomach even if the drug is predominantly ionized in the intestine and largely nonionized in the stomach. Thus, any factor that accelerates gastric emptying (recumbent position right side) will generally increase the rate of drug absorption, whereas any factor that delays gastric emptying will have the opposite effect. The gastric emptying rate is influenced by numerous factors, including the caloric content of food; volume, osmolality, temperature, and pH of ingested fluid; diurnal and interindividual variation; metabolic state (rest or exercise); and the ambient temperature. Gastric emptying is influenced in women by the effects of estrogen (i.e. compared to men, emptying is slower for premenopausal women and those taking estrogen replacement therapy).

Drugs that are destroyed by gastric secretions and low pH or that cause gastric irritation sometimes are administered in dosage forms with an enteric coating that prevents dissolution in the acidic gastric contents. Enteric coatings are useful for drugs that can cause gastric irritation and for presenting a drug such as mesalamine to sites of action in the ileum and colon.

2. Match the following drugs with their ocular adverse effects?

Drugs	Adverse effects
1. Amiodarone	A. Blepharoconjunctivitis
2. Hydroxychloroquine	B. Angle closure glaucoma
3. Systemic steroids	C. Retinopathy
4. Digoxin	D. Optic neuritis
	E. Yellow vision
	F. Cataract
	G. Corneal microdeposits

Ans. 1-G, 2-C, 3-F, 4-E

Ocular Side Effects of Systemic Agents

Glaucoma

The antiseizure drug topiramate can cause choroidal effusions leading to angle-closure glaucoma.

Retina

- Hydroxychloroquine and chloroquine can cause central retinal toxicity by an unknown mechanism. With normal dosages, toxicity does not appear until about 6 years after the drug is started. Stopping the drug will not reverse the damage but generally will prevent further toxicity.
- Tamoxifen can cause crystalline maculopathy.

- Vigabatrin causes progressive and permanent bilateral concentric visual field constriction in a high percentage of patients.
- Digoxin can cause altered color perception and coronas (halos).

Optic Nerve

- The PDE5 inhibitors sildenafil, vardenafil, and tadalafil inhibit PDE5 in the corpus cavernosum to help achieve and maintain penile erection and to treat pulmonary arterial hypertension.
- Multiple medications, including ethambutol, chloramphenicol, and rifampin, can cause toxic optic neuropathy characterized by gradually progressive bilateral central scotomas and vision loss.
- Systemic or ocular steroids can cause elevated IOP and glaucoma. If the steroids cannot be stopped, glaucoma medications, and even filtering surgery, often are required.

Anterior Segment

- Steroids and tamoxifen have been implicated in cataract formation.
- Rifabutin, if used in conjunction with clarithromycin or fluconazole for treatment of Mycobacterium avium complex opportunistic infections in HIV-positive persons, is associated with an iridocyclitis and even hypopyon.

Ocular Surface

- Isotretinoin has a drying effect on mucous membranes and is associated with dry eye and severe dysfunction of the meibomian gland.

Cornea, Conjunctiva, and Eyelids

- One of the most common drug deposits found in the cornea is from the cardiac medication amiodarone. It deposits in the inferior and central cornea in a whorl-like pattern termed cornea verticillata, appearing as fine tan or brown pigment in the epithelium. The deposits seldom affect vision and are rarely a cause to discontinue the medication. The deposits disappear slowly when the medication is stopped.
- Other medications, including indomethacin, atovaquone, chloroquine, and hydroxychloroquine, can cause a similar pattern.
- The phenothiazines, including chlorpromazine and thioridazine, can cause brown pigmentary deposits in the cornea, conjunctiva, and eyelids. They typically do not affect vision. The ocular deposits generally persist after discontinuation of the medication and can even worsen.
- Tetracyclines can cause a yellow discoloration of the light-exposed conjunctiva.
- Systemic minocycline can induce a blue-gray scleral pigmentation that is most prominent in the interpalpebral zone.

3. Propranolol is drug of choice for?

a. Ulcerated infantile hemangioma
b. Lymphangioma
c. Pyogenic granuloma
d. Capillary malformation

Ans. a. Ulcerated infantile hemangioma

Propranolol

Pharmacological actions

- Heart rate reduces
- Reduced contractility
- Reduced cardiac output
- Slow conduction in atria and AV node
- Prolonged refractory period, AV node
- Bronchoconstriction
- Prolonged hypoglycemia
- Reduced plasma levels of free fatty acids
- Increased plasma levels of HDL cholesterol
- Raised LDL cholesterol and triglycerides
- Hypokalemia

Clinical uses

- Angina pectoris
- Hypertension
- Cardiac arrhythmias
- Congestive heart failure
- Pheochromocytoma
- Glaucoma
- Hypertrophic obstructive cardiomyopathy
- Hyperthyroidism
- Migraine prophylaxis
- Acute panic symptoms
- Substance abuse withdrawal
- Infantile hemangioma
- Variceal bleeding in portal hypertension

Adverse effects

- Bradycardia
- Negative inotropy
- Reduced cardiac output
- Bradyarrhythmias
- Slowing of AV conduction resulting in AV block
- Bronchoconstriction
- Fatigue
- Sleep disturbances (insomnia, nightmares)

- Prolongation of hypoglycemia
- Sexual dysfunction in men

4. Preferred drug for the treatment of uncomplicated grade 2 hypertension in a 48-year-old man is:

a. Chlorthalidone
b. Triamterene
c. Spironolactone
d. Furosemide

Ans. a. Chlorthalidone

Thiazide Diuretics

Various thiazide and related diuretics include: Bendroflumethiazide, Chlorothiazide, Chlorthalidone, Hydrochlorothiazide, Hydroflumethiazide, Indapamide, Methyclothiazide, Metolazone, Polythiazide, Quinethazone, Trichlormethiazide.

Pharmacodynamics

Thiazides inhibit NaCl reabsorption from the luminal side of epithelial cells in the DCT by blocking the Na^+/Cl^- transporter (NCC). In contrast to the situation in the TAL, in which loop diuretics inhibit Ca^{2+} reabsorption, thiazides actually enhance Ca^{2+} reabsorption. This enhancement has been postulated to result from effects in both the proximal and distal convoluted tubules. In the proximal tubule, thiazide-induced volume depletion leads to enhanced N^{a+} and passive Ca^{2+} reabsorption. In the DCT, lowering of intracellular Na^+ by thiazide-induced blockade of Na^+ entry enhances Na^+/Ca^{2+} exchange in the basolateral membrane and increases overall reabsorption of Ca^{2+}. Although thiazides rarely cause hypercalcemia as a result of this enhanced reabsorption, they can unmask hypercalcemia due to other causes (e.g., primary hyperparathyroidism, carcinoma, sarcoidosis). Thiazides are sometimes useful in the prevention of calcium-containing kidney stones caused by hypercalciuria. They may also modestly reduce the risk of osteoporotic fractures.

The action of thiazides depends in part on renal prostaglandin production. As described for loop diuretics, the actions of thiazides can also be inhibited by NSAIDs under certain conditions.

Clinical Indications and Dosage

The major indications for thiazide diuretics are (1) hypertension, (2) heart failure, (3) nephrolithiasis due to idiopathic hypercalciuria, and (4) nephrogenic diabetes insipidus. Thiazide diuretics are inexpensive, are generally well tolerated, and are recommended as a first-line therapy in the treatment of hypertension in the elderly population.

Toxicity

A. Hypokalemic metabolic alkalosis
B. Impaired carbohydrate tolerance

C. Hyperlipidemia
D. Hyponatremia
E. Impaired uric acid metabolism and gout
F. Allergic reactions.

5. Mention the true/false statements about digoxin toxicity?

a. Earliest manifestation of digoxin toxicity are gastrointestinal symptoms
b. Nonspecific vision changes may be noted in digoxin toxicity
c. Early toxicity may not correlate with serum levels
d. Neurological symptoms may occur without corresponding cardiovascular changes
e. None

Ans. a-T, b-T, c-T, d-T

Adverse Effects of Digoxin

The therapeutic index of digoxin is extremely narrow, about 2: plasma concentrations between 0.5 and 0.8 ng/mL are associated with beneficial effects, and concentrations of 1.2 ng/mL and greater are associated with a tendency toward increased mortality. The most frequent and most serious adverse effects are arrhythmias. In digoxin overdosing, patients exhibit arrhythmias (90%), GI symptoms (~55%), and neurotoxic symptoms (~12%). The most frequent causes of toxicity are renal insufficiency and overdosing.

The classic digoxin effect appears as a downsloping ST segment depression with T inversion, also known as the "reverse tick" or "reverse check" sign. PR interval prolongation can also be seen, due to direct vagomimetic slowing effect on AV node. Cardiac toxicity in healthy persons presents as extreme bradycardia, atrial fibrillation, and AV block, whereas ventricular arrhythmias are rare. In patients with structural heart disease, frequent signs of digoxin toxicity are ventricular extrasystoles, bigeminy, ventricular tachycardia, and fibrillation. In principle, however, every type of arrhythmia can be CG induced. GI adverse effects are anorexia, nausea, and vomiting, mainly as a result of digoxin effects on chemosensors in the area postrema. Spastic contraction of the mesenteric artery can rarely lead to severe diarrhea and life-threatening necrosis of the intestine. Headache, fatigue, and sleeplessness can be early symptoms of CG toxicity. Typical, albeit not too common (10%), are visual effects: altered color perception and coronas (halos).

Treatment

Cessation of CG medication normally suffices as therapy of CG toxicity. However, severe arrhythmias, such as extreme bradycardia or complex ventricular arrhythmias, require active therapy.

Extreme sinus bradycardia, sinoatrial block, or AV block grade II or III: Atropine (0.5–1 mg) IV. If not successful, a temporary pacemaker may be necessary.

Tachycardiac ventricular arrhythmias and hypokalemia: K^+ infusion (40–60 mmol/d). Consider that high K^+ can aggravate AV conduction defects.

An effective antidote for digoxin toxicity is antidigoxin immunotherapy. Purified Fab fragments from ovine antidigoxin antisera (Digibind) are usually dosed by the estimated total dose of digoxin ingested to achieve a fully neutralizing effect.

6. A bank employee suffering from depression came to AIIMS OPD. He was started on Escitalopram. Which of these adverse effects cannot be explained with escitalopram?

a. Vivid dreaming
b. Anorgasmia
c. Sialorrhea
d. Nausea

Ans. c. Sialorrhea

Side Effects of Antidepressants

Tricyclic antidepressants

- Anticholinergic effects—dry mouth, constipation, urinary retention (especially in elderly men with BPH), blurred vision, palpitation.
- Sedation and tinnitus are common.
- Weight gain and increased appetite
- Patients with bipolar disorder may develop manic episode on starting treatment.
- Sweating and fine tremors are relatively common.
- They may lower seizure threshold precipitating convulsions.
- Postural hypotension, especially in older patients
- Cardiac arrhythmias may occur, especially in patients with ischemic heart disease.
- Rashes and jaundice due to hypersensitivity are rare.

SSRIs and SNRIs

- *GI side effects*: Nausea, vomiting, diarrhea (because of increased serotonergic tone in GIT)
- *Sexual side effects*: Diminished sexual function and interest, leading to loss of libido, delayed orgasm/ anorgasmia or diminished arousal (because of increased serotonergic tone at the level of spinal cord and above).
- *Others*: Headache, insomnia/ hypersomnia, irritability, weight gain, dizziness, Paresthesia etc. They can also lead to vivid dreams.
- Discontinuation syndrome can occur with shorter acting SSRIs like paroxetine and sertraline.

7. Chlorpromazine acts on which of the following receptors?

1. D2 and 5HT2 receptors
2. GABA and Beta-adrenergic receptors
3. Muscarinic M1 and alpha-adrenergic receptors

4. H1 receptors
a. 1, 3 and 4 are correct
b. Only 2 is correct
c. 1 and 2 are correct
d. All are correct

Ans. a. 1, 3 and 4 are correct

Chlorpromazine

Chlorpromazine is a psychotropic agent indicated for the treatment of schizophrenia. It also exerts sedative and antiemetic activity.

Chlorpromazine has actions at all levels of the central nervous system—primarily at subcortical levels—as well as on multiple organ systems.

Chlorpromazine has strong antiadrenergic and weaker peripheral anticholinergic activity; ganglionic blocking action is relatively slight.

It also possesses slight antihistaminic and antiserotonin activity.

Traditional antipsychotic agent with anti-emetic activity.

Mechanism of action

Exerts its antipsychotic effect by blocking postsynaptic dopamine receptors in cortical and limbic areas of the brain, thereby preventing the excess of dopamine in the brain.

This leads to a reduction in psychotic symptoms, such as hallucinations and delusions.

Chlorpromazine appears to exert its anti-emetic activity by blocking dopamine receptors in the chemical trigger zone (CTZ) in the brain, thereby relieving nausea and vomiting.

8. Most commonly implicated drug for acute liver failure is:

a. Paracetamol
b. Valproate
c. Warfarin
d. Tetracyclines

Ans. a. Paracetamol

Paracetamol

Paracetamol is the active metabolite of phenacetin and is responsible for its analgesic effect. It is a weak COX-1 and COX-2 inhibitor in peripheral tissues and possesses no significant anti-inflammatory effects.

Pharmacokinetics: Acetaminophen is administered orally. Acetaminophen is poorly bound to plasma proteins and is partially metabolized by hepatic microsomal enzymes to the inactive sulfate and glucuronide. In large doses, a minor but highly reactive metabolite (N-acetyl-p-benzoquinone) is important because it is toxic to both liver and kidney.

The half-life of acetaminophen is 2–3 hours and is relatively unaffected by renal function. With toxic doses or liver disease, the half-life may be increased twofold or more.

Indications: Although said to be equivalent to aspirin as an analgesic and antipyretic agent, acetaminophen lacks anti-inflammatory properties. It does not affect uric acid levels and lacks platelet-inhibiting effects. The drug is useful in mild to moderate pain such as headache, myalgia, postpartum pain, and other circumstances in which aspirin is an effective analgesic. Acetaminophen alone is inadequate therapy for inflammatory conditions such as RA. For mild analgesia, acetaminophen is the preferred drug in patients allergic to aspirin, when salicylates are poorly tolerated. It is preferable to aspirin in patients with hemophilia, in those with a history of peptic ulcer, and in those in whom bronchospasm is precipitated by aspirin. Unlike aspirin, acetaminophen does not antagonize the effects of uricosuric agents.

Adverse effects: In therapeutic doses, a mild reversible increase in hepatic enzymes may occasionally occur. With larger doses, dizziness, excitement, and disorientation may occur. Ingestion of 15 g of acetaminophen may be fatal, death being caused by severe hepatotoxicity with centrilobular necrosis, sometimes associated with acute renal tubular necrosis.

Present data indicate that even 4 g acetaminophen is associated with increased liver function test abnormalities. Doses greater than 4 g/d are not usually recommended, and a history of alcoholism contraindicates even this dose. Early symptoms of hepatic damage include nausea, vomiting, diarrhea, and abdominal pain. Cases of renal damage without hepatic damage have occurred, even after usual doses of acetaminophen. Therapy for overdose is much less satisfactory than that for aspirin overdose. In addition to supportive therapy, one should provide sulfhydryl groups in the form of acetylcysteine to neutralize the toxic metabolites.

Hemolytic anemia and methemoglobinemia are very rare adverse events. Interstitial nephritis and papillary necrosis—serious complications of phenacetin—have not occurred, and GI bleeding also has not occurred. Caution is necessary in patients with any type of liver disease.

Dosage: Acute pain and fever may be effectively treated with 325–500 mg four times daily and proportionately less for children. Dosing in adults is now recommended not to exceed 4 g/d, in most cases.

9. Which of the following is/are adverse effect of SGLT2 inhibitors?

1. Ketoacidosis	a. 1, 2 and 4 are correct
2. Urosepsis	b. 1, 2 and 3 are correct

3. Fournier's gangrene
4. Angioedema

c. Only 4 is correct
d. All are correct

Ans. b. 1, 2 and 3 are correct

Sodium glucose co-transporter-2 inhibitors (SGLT-2 inhibitors): Glucose is freely filtered by the renal glomeruli and is reabsorbed in the proximal tubules by the action of sodium-glucose transporters (SGLTs). Sodium-glucose transporter 2 (SGLT2) accounts for 90% of glucose reabsorption, and its inhibition causes glycosuria and lowers glucose levels in patients with type 2 diabetes. SGLT2 inhibitors lower glucose levels by changing the renal threshold and not by insulin action. The SGLT2 inhibitors canagliflozin, dapagliflozin, and empagliflozin, all oral medications, are approved for clinical use.

Side effects: Ketoacidosis, urosepsis, Fournier's gangrene, increased incidence of UTI & genital infections.

10. Clostridium difficile diarrhea is most commonly associated with?

a. Aminopenicillins
b. Fluoroquinolones
c. Macrolides
d. Carbapenems

Ans. a. Aminopenicillins

C. difficile is an obligately anaerobic, gram-positive, spore-forming bacillus whose spores are found widely in nature, particularly in the environment of hospitals and chronic-care facilities. *C. difficile* occurs frequently in hospitals and nursing homes (or shortly after discharge from these facilities) where the level of antimicrobial use is high and the environment is contaminated by *C. difficile* spores.

Clindamycin, ampicillin, and cephalosporins were the first antibiotics associated with *C. difficile*. The aminopenicillins and second - and third-generation cephalosporins, particularly cefotaxime, ceftriaxone, cefuroxime, and ceftazidime, are agents frequently responsible for this condition. The fluoroquinolones (ciprofloxacin, levofloxacin, and moxifloxacin) are the most recent drug class to be implicated in hospital outbreaks. Penicillin/β-lactamase-inhibitor combinations such as ticarcillin/clavulanate and piperacillin/tazobactam pose significantly less risk. However, all antibiotics, including vancomycin and metronidazole (the agents most commonly used to treat *C. difficile*), have been found to carry a risk of subsequent *C. difficile*. A few cases, especially in the community, are reported in patients without documentation of prior antibiotic exposure.

11. During the investigation for an outbreak of MRSA in the hospital, it was found that a nurse of NICU had MRSA colonization of anterior nares. What is the best treatment for her?

a. Topical bacitracin
b. Oral vancomycin
c. Inhaled colistin
d. IV cefazolin

Ans. **a. Topical bacitracin**

Management of Skin Infections Caused by *Staph. aureus*

Topical treatment includes mupirocin applied three times daily to the involved skin and nares, as approximately 25% of people are carriers of *S. aureus*. Although treatment helps reduce autoinoculation and communicable spread, treatment also contributes to the growing resistance of *S. aureus* against mupirocin. Because mupirocin is a cornerstone of MRSA treatment, many authors recommend it be reserved for MRSA carriers with recurrent infections only. Although a 1- or 2-week course of mupirocin may not be enough time for the emergence of resistant strains, prolonged treatment with mupirocin is not advised for chronic conditions.

Retapamulin 1% ointment applied twice daily for 5 days is an effective alternative to mupirocin. To eliminate staphylococcal carriage in impetigo patients, rifampin and dicloxacillin are often used, as well as the topical antiseptics polyhexanide, polyvidone, octenidine, and chlorhexidine. CA-MRSA in impetigo is increasingly common in the pediatric population, and treatment includes clindamycin, trimethoprim-sulfamethoxazole, tetracycline, and fluoroquinolones.

12. Fixed drug eruptions are frequently seen with?

a. Penicillin
b. Sulfonamide
c. Cetirizine
d. Roxithromycin

Ans. **b. Sulfonamide**

Drugs causing fixed drug eruptions:

- Paracetamol (Phenacetin)
- Sulfonamides
- NSAIDs
- Aspirin
- Barbiturates
- Dapsone
- Tetracyclines
- Phenylbutazone

13. Assertion: Large doses of acyclovir are recommended for treating genital herpes in HIV positive patients
Reason: Frequent recurrence of genital herpes is seen in HIV patients:

a. Both Assertion and Reason are true and Reason is correct explanation of Assertion
b. Assertion is true & reason is not the right explanation for assertion
c. Assertion is false & reason is also false
d. Both assertion & reason are false
e. Both Assertion and Reason are independently a false/incorrect statement

Ans. **a. Both Assertion and Reason are true and Reason is correct explanation of Assertion**

Acyclovir

Mechanism of action:

Acyclovir requires three phosphorylation steps for activation. It is converted first to the monophosphate derivative by the virus-specified thymidine kinase and then to the di- and triphosphate compounds by host cell enzymes. Because it requires the viral kinase for initial phosphorylation, acyclovir is selectively activated—and the active metabolite accumulates—only in infected cells. Acyclovir triphosphate inhibits viral DNA synthesis by two mechanisms: competition with deoxyGTP for the viral DNA polymerase, resulting in binding to the DNA template as an irreversible complex; and chain termination following incorporation into the viral DNA.

Therapeutic uses

Acyclovir's clinical use is limited to herpesviruses. Acyclovir is most active against HSV-1, approximately half as active against HSV-2, a tenth as potent against VZV and EBV, and least active against CMV and HHV-6.

In immunocompetent persons, the clinical benefits of acyclovir and valacyclovir are greater in initial HSV infections than in recurrent ones. These drugs are particularly useful in immunocompromised patients because these individuals experience both more frequent and more severe HSV and VZV infections. Because VZV is less susceptible than HSV to acyclovir, higher doses must be used for treating VZV infections. Oral valacyclovir is as effective as oral acyclovir in HSV infections and more effective for treating herpes zoster. Acyclovir is ineffective therapeutically in established CMV infections, but ganciclovir is effective for CMV prophylaxis in immunocompromised patients. EBV-related oral hairy leukoplakia may improve with acyclovir. Oral acyclovir in conjunction with systemic corticosteroids appears beneficial in treating Bell palsy; valacyclovir is ineffective in acute vestibular neuritis.

14. Mention the true/false statements about drug resistant malaria?

a. Not present in India
b. Quinine with clindamycin or doxycycline is still effective treatment
c. Chloroquine with sulfadoxine-pyrimethamine is effective
d. Artemether with lumefantrine is useful
e. Monotherapy with artemisinin derivatives is not useful due to high relapse rate

Ans. a-F, b-T, c-F, d-T, e-T

Multidrug resistance of *P. Falciparum* is seen when the parasite is resistant to more than two operational antimalarial compounds of different chemical classes and modes of action.

Generally, the two classes first affected are the 4-aminoquinolines and the antifolates (diaminopyrimidine, sulfonamides).

Drug resistance results in a delay in or failure to clear asexual parasites from the blood, which allows production of the gametocytes that are responsible for transmission of the resistant genotype.

Drug Resistance in India

In India, chloroquine-resistant *P. falciparum* malaria has been observed with increasing frequency across the country in recent years.

Considering this, the Government of India has recommended the combination of artesunate and Sulfa-Pyrimethamine as the treatment of choice for *P. falciparum* (and mixed) infections all across the country.

In north east India, where resistance to SP has been documented, the National Drug Policy recommends the use of Artemether and Lumefantrine for the treatment of *P. falciparum* malaria. *P. vivax* remains sensitive to chloroquine all across the country.

15. Match the following drugs with organism they are used for:

Drugs:	Organisms:
1. Praziquantel	A. Filaria
2. Diethylcarbamazine	B. Giardia
3. Nitazoxanide	C. Strongyloides
4. Mebendazole	D. Tapeworms
	E. Leishmania
	F. Ascaris lumbricoides

Ans. 1-D, 2-A, 3-B, 4-F

Anthelmintic Drugs

Drugs	Therapeutic uses
Albendazole	➤ Intestinal nematode infections ➤ Cysticercosis ➤ Cutaneous larva migrans ➤ Toxocariasis ➤ Echinococcosis
Mebendazole	➤ Intestinal nematode infections
Triclabendazole	➤ Fascioliasis
Ivermectin	➤ Onchocerciasis ➤ Lymphatic filariasis ➤ Scabies and head lice ➤ Strongyloidiasis
Praziquental	➤ Schistosomiasis ➤ Food-borne trematode infections (opisthorciasis and paragonamiasis) ➤ Intestinal tapeworm infections
Diethylcarbamazine	➤ Lymphatic filariasis
Metrifonate	➤ Second-line drug for *Schistosoma haematobium* infection
Oxamniquine	➤ Second-line drug for *Schistosoma mansoni* infection
Niclosamide	➤ Intestinal tapeworm infection
Oxantel and pyrantel pamoate	➤ Second-line drug for intestinal nematode infection
Doxycycline	➤ Filarial infection
Levamisole	➤ Excellent activity against *Ascaris lumbricoides* ➤ Low-to-moderate efficacy against *Trichuris trichiura* and hookworm infections
Nitazoxanide	➤ Effective against intestinal helminths ➤ Antiprotozoal and antiviral activity

16. What is the mechanism of action of deferoxamine when given for the treatment of iron poisoning?

a. Binding with trivalent Fe^{3+}
b. Inhibiting Hepcidin
c. Inhibiting DMT1
d. Inhibiting ferroportin

Ans. **a. Binding with trivalent Fe^{3+}**

Deferoxamine

Deferoxamine is a specific chelating agent for iron. It binds free iron and, to some extent, loosely bound ferric iron (e.g., from ferritin or hemosiderin). Iron bound to hemoglobin, transferrin, cytochrome enzymes, and all other sites is not affected. The red iron-deferoxamine (ferrioxamine) complex is water-soluble and excreted renally; it may impart an orange-pink (vin rose) color to the urine. Deferasirox is a newer tridentate chelator with selectively high affinity for iron.

Clinical Use

Deferoxamine is used parenterally in the treatment of acute iron intoxication and in the treatment of iron overload caused by blood transfusions in patients with diseases such as thalassemia or myelodysplastic syndrome. Deferasirox is an oral drug approved for treatment of iron overload.

Toxicity

Skin reactions (blushing, erythema, urticaria) may occur. With long-term use, neurotoxicity (e.g., retinal degeneration), hepatic and renal dysfunction, and severe coagulopathies have been reported. Rapid intravenous administration of deferoxamine can cause histamine release and hypotensive shock.

Microbiology

1. Mark the following statements regarding malaria as true or false:

a. Black water fever is caused by *P. ovale*
b. Cerebral malaria is caused by *P. falciparum*
c. Duffy antigen offers protection against *P. vivax*
d. Sickle cell anemia aggravates *P falciparum* malaria
e. None

Ans. **a–F, b–T, c–F, d–F**

Manifestations of Severe Falciparum Malaria

Signs	Manifestations
Major	
Unarousable coma/cerebral malaria	Failure to localize or respond appropriately to noxious stimuli; coma persisting for >30 min after generalized convulsion
Acidemia/acidosis	Arterial pH of <7.25, base deficit >8 mEq/L, or plasma bicarbonate level of <15 mmol/L; venous lactate level of >5 mmol/L; manifests as labored deep breathing, often termed "respiratory distress"
Severe normochromic, normocytic anemia	Hematocrit of <15% or hemoglobin level of <50 g/L (<5 g/dL) with parasitemia level of <10,000/μL
Renal failure	Serum or plasma creatinine level of >265 μmol/L (>3 mg/dL); urine output (24 h) of <400 mL for adults or <12 mL/kg for children; no improvement with rehydration
Pulmonary edema/adult respiratory distress syndrome	Noncardiogenic pulmonary edema, often aggravated by overhydration
Hypoglycemia	Plasma glucose level of <2.2 mmol/L (<40 mg/dL)
Hypotension/shock	Systolic blood pressure of <50 mm Hg in children 1–5 years or <80 mm Hg in adults; core/skin temperature difference of >10°C; capillary refill >2 s
Bleeding/disseminated intravascular coagulation	Significant bleeding and hemorrhage from the gums, nose, and gastrointestinal tract and/or evidence of disseminated intravascular coagulation
Convulsions	More than two generalized seizures in 24 h; signs of continued seizure activity, sometimes subtle (e.g., tonic-clonic eye movements without limb or face movement)

Contd…

Contd...

Signs	Manifestations
Other	
Hemoglobinuria (Black water fever)	Macroscopic black, brown, or red urine; not associated with effects of oxidant drugs and red blood cell enzyme defects (such as G6PD deficiency)
Extreme weakness	Prostration; inability to sit unaided
Hyperparasitemia	Parasitemia level of >5% in nonimmune patients (>10% in any patient)
Jaundice	Serum bilirubin level of >50 mmol/L (>3 mg/dL) if combined with a parasite density of 100,000/μL or other evidence of vital-organ dysfunction

The Duffy blood-group antigen Fya or Fyb plays an important role in invasion. Individuals who carry the Duffy-negative FyFy phenotype are generally resistant to *P. vivax* malaria. *P. knowlesi* also invades Duffy-positive human RBCs preferentially.

The possession of the sickle cell allele protects these individuals against malaria because the parasite dies when potassium leaks out of RBCs as they become sickle shaped.

Types of anemia that have protective effect against *P. falciparum* malaria are—G6PD deficiency, Sickle cell anemia, Thalassemia, HbC, Pyruvate kinase deficiency.

2. Components of the Ziehl-Neelsen stain used for cryptosporidium are:

a. Carbol fuschin
b. Methylene blue
c. Iodine
d. Malachite green
e. None

Ans. a–T, b–T, c–F, d–F

The Acid-fast Stain (ZN stain)

Acid fastness is a property of the mycobacteria (e.g., Mycobacterium tuberculosis) and related organisms. Acid-fast organisms generally stain very poorly with dyes, including those used in the Gram stain. However, they can be stained by prolonged application of more concentrated dyes, by penetrating agents, or by heat treatment. Their unique feature is that when stained, acid-fast bacteria resist decolorization by concentrations of mineral acids and ethanol that remove the same dyes from other bacteria. This combination of weak initial staining and strong retention once stained is related to the high lipid content of the mycobacterial cell wall. Acid-fast stains are completed with a counterstain to provide a contrasting background for viewing the stained bacteria.

In the acid-fast procedure, the slide is flooded with carbol-fuchsin (red) and decolorized with hydrochloric acid in alcohol. When counter-stained with methylene blue, acid-fast organisms appear red against a blue background. A variant is the fluorochrome stain, which uses a fluorescent dye (auramine, or an auramine–rhodamine mixture), followed by decolorization with acid–alcohol. Acid-fast organisms retain the fluorescent stain, which allows their visualization by fluorescence microscopy.

3. A patient presented with a rash as given in the image. This condition is associated with which of the following professions?

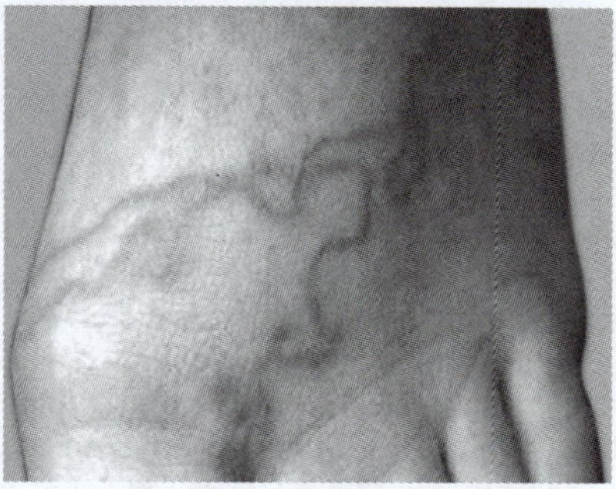

a. Swimming pool staff
b. Dog kennel cleaner
c. Butcher
d. Poultry worker

Ans. b. Dog kennel cleaner

Larva Migrans

- It is caused as a result of entry of non-human nematodes into the human body. They tend to wander around aimlessly within various tissues of the body, causing inflammation. It is of 2 types:

Cutaneous Larva Migrans

- Also called creeping eruption, it is caused by non-human nematode larvae entering the human body by skin penetration.
- Serpiginous tunnels are formed in the epidermis as a result of the migration, producing itchy lesions.
- It is called creeping eruption due the shifting nature of lesions in accordance with the movement of the larva.
- It is most commonly caused by Ancylostoma braziliense and A. caninum
- *Treatment*: Thiabendazole.

Visceral Larva Migrans

- It is caused by migration of larvae of non-human nematodes into visceral organs.

- They usually enter through the intestinal tract, following which they penetrate the mucosa and travel into various organs aimlessly causing inflammation.
- Most commonly caused by Toxocaracanis and T. cati.

4. Identify the correct sequence in which the following agents are applied during Gram's stain procedure:

a. Iodine b. Safranin red
c. Carbol fuchsin d. Gentian violet

Ans. d: Gentian violet, a: Iodine, c: Carbol fuchsin, b: Safranin red

Procedure of Gram's Stain

- *Application of the primary stain* (crystal violet/Gentian violet): It stains the cells as blue/purple
- *Application of a mordant*: The iodine solution is used as a mordant, which combines with the stain to fix it within the cells. It is added to form a crystal violet-iodine complex; all cells continue to appear blue.
- *Decolorization*: This step helps in distinguishing gram-positive from gram-negative cells. The organic solvent such as acetone or ethanol, extracts the blue dye complex from the lipid-rich, thin-walled gram-negative bacteria to a greater degree than from the lipid-poor, thick-walled, gram-positive bacteria. The gram-negative bacteria appear colorless and gram-positive bacteria remain blue.
- *Application of counterstain*: The counterstain- safranin stains the decolorized gram-negative cells red/pink; the gram-positive bacteria remain blue.

5. A patient presented with fever for 8 days and difficulty in breathing for two days, on examination there is red painless rash found on the left side of the chest. What is the most likely diagnosis?

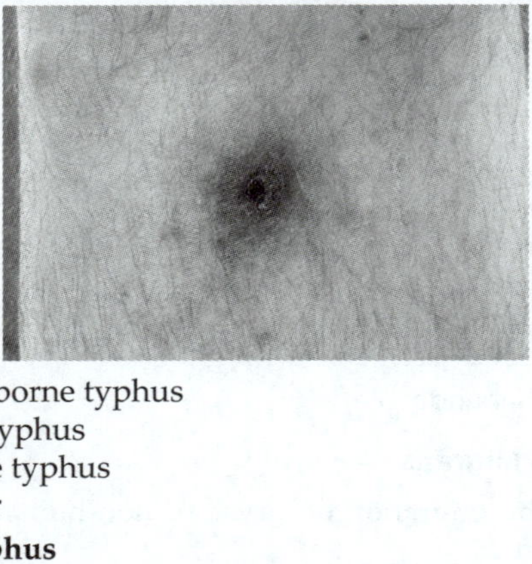

a. Louse-borne typhus
b. Scrub typhus
c. Murine typhus
d. Q fever

Ans. b. Scrub typhus

Rickettsial Infections

Disease	Agent	Insect vector	Mammalian reservoir
1. Typhus group a. Epidemic typhus b. Murine typhus (Endemic typhus) c. Scrub typhus	R. prowazekii R. typhi R. tsutsugamushi	Louse Flea Mite	Humans Rodents Rodents
2. Spotted fever group a. Indian tick typhus b. Rocky mountain spotted fever c. Rickettsial pox	R. conori R rickettsii R akari	Tick Tick Mite	Rodents, dogs Rodents, dogs Mice
3. Others a. Q fever b. Trench fever	C burnetii Bartonella quintana	Nil Louse	Cattle, sheep, goats Humans

Scrub Typhus

- It is a form of typhus caused by Orientia tsutsugamushi first isolated and identified in 1930 in Japan
- Scrub typhus is transmitted by some species of trombiculid mites ("chiggers", particularly Leptotrombidium deliense), which are found in areas of heavy scrub vegetation.
- The bite of this mite leaves a characteristic black eschar that is useful for making the diagnosis.
- Scrub typhus is endemic to a part of the world known as the "tsutsugamushi triangle" (after the name "Orientia tsutsugamushi" (formerly "Rickettsia tsutsugamushi").

Treatment

- Doxycycline is the drug of choice for rickettsia.
- Azithromycin, fluoroquinolones and chloramphenicol are other alternatives.

6. Which among the following exist in yeast form at 37°C and hyphal form at 25°C?

a. Malassezia furfur
b. Cryptococcus neoformans
c. Aspergillus
d. Histoplasma capsulatum

Ans. **d. Histoplasma capsulatum**

Classification of Fungi

Genus	Typical growth	Septation	Phylum
Superficial Fungi			
Epidermophyton	Mold	+	Ascomycota
Microsporum	Mold	+	Ascomycota
Trichophyton	Mold	+	Ascomycota
Subcutaneous Fungi			
Sporothrix	Dimorphic	+	Ascomycota
Opportunistic Fungi			
Aspergillus	Mold	+	Ascomycota
Candida	Dimorphic	+	Ascomycota
Mucor	Mold	-	Zygomycota
Pneumocystis	Cysts		Ascomycota
Rhizopus	Mold	-	Zygomycota
Systemic Fungi			
Blastomyces	Dimorphic	+	Ascomycota
Coccidioides	Dimorphic	+	Ascomycota
Cryptococcus	Yeast		Basidiomycota
Histoplasma	Dimorphic	+	Ascomycota

Dimorphism

- Although many fungi tend to grow as either yeasts or molds, some species can transition between morphological forms depending on environmental conditions. These species are known as dimorphic fungi. Many fungi, including the most common human fungal pathogen *Candida albicans*, display a striking ability to modify their cellular shape and structure in order to adapt to new environments. These morphological transitions are often very important for the pathogenesis of human infections.
- A distinct group of human pathogens are the thermally dimorphic fungi, shifting from yeast-like to hyphal growth based on temperature. These fungal species tend to grow in the mold form in their environmental reservoir as well as when incubated in culture at ambient temperatures. However, they convert to a yeast-like growth form in the mammalian host or when incubated in culture at 37°C. For most, it is possible to manipulate the culture conditions to demonstrate both yeast and mold phases *in vitro*. Yeast phase growth requires conditions similar to those of the physiologic *in vivo* environment, such as 35°C to 37°C incubation and enriched medium. Mold growth requires minimal nutrients and ambient temperatures. Importantly, the conidia produced in the mold phase may be infectious and serve to disseminate the fungus during growth in the environment.

7. Medlar bodies are found in:

a. Chromoblastomycosis
b. Sporotrichosis
c. Mycetoma
d. Candidiasis

Ans. a. Chromoblastomycosis

Chromoblastomycosis

Chromoblastomycosis is a chronic form of skin infection caused by multiple species of pigmented saprophytic fungi, also known as melanized or "dematiaceous" fungi. Disease caused by Fonsecaea, Phialophora, and Cladophialophora (Cladosporium) species typically occurs on the foot or leg, the sites of skin inoculation by the fungus. Primary lesions appear as papules that develop into scaly, wart-like structures, usually under the feet. Fully developed lesions have been likened to the tips of a cauliflower. Extension occurs through painless, slowly progressive satellite lesions. The organisms are found in the soil of endemic areas, and most infections occur in individuals who work barefoot. Disseminated infections due to the dematiaceous molds are uncommon, observed almost exclusively in highly immunocompromised patients. In fact, in these patients certain pigmented molds have a predilection for infecting the central nervous system. Therefore, in highly immunocompromised patients, the isolation of a pigmented mold from a clinical specimen cannot necessarily be ignored as a contaminant.

The outstanding mycologic feature in chromoblastomycosis is the presence in histological sections of brown-pigmented, thick-walled, multiseptate, 5 to 12 mm globose structures called muriform bodies, sclerotic bodies, Medlar bodies or copper-penny cells. Branching septate hyphae may also be demonstrated in KOH preparations of tissue scrapings. In culture, these fungi grow as darkly pigmented molds. Surgery and antifungal therapy have been used in chromoblastomycosis, but cure rates of advanced disease are disappointing. Flucytosine or itraconazole are the systemic antifungal agents most frequently used for this infection.

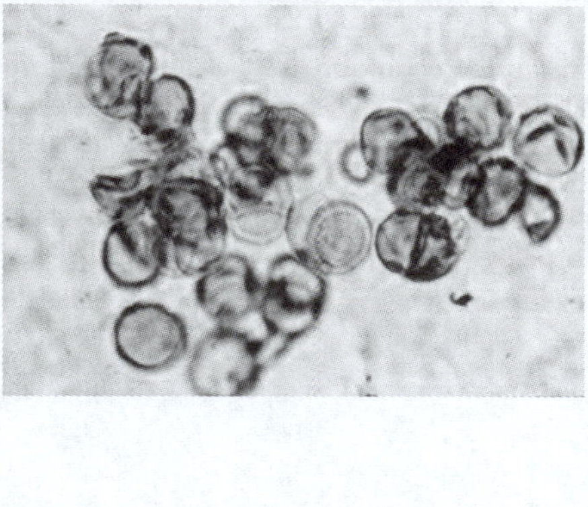

8. Mark the following statements regarding xenodiagnoses as true or false:

a. Blood from suspected dengue patient can be used for cultivation in Aedes mosquito
b. Effect on rabbit ileal loop is used for diagnosis of ETEC
c. Coxiella is cultivated in eggs synthesise antigen required for antibody detection
d. Sandfly can be grown in Hamster eggs

Ans. a–T, b–T, c–T, d–F

Xenodiagnosis

A method for diagnosing a disease in one organism by inoculating the putative causative organism in a second animal of a different species. It has been used for the detection of parasites when peripheral blood smears are negative.

Various examples are

- *Sandfly*: Only female sand flies take a blood meal. The females need the proteins present in the blood to lay eggs and to propagate the future generation. Various blood meal sources can be used depending on the availability of source animals and the preference of the flies. It may be necessary to try several blood-meal sources and feeding times until a suitable host and feeding time is found. Routinely used organisms are mice, hamsters and nude guinea pigs.
- *Dengue virus*: Intra-thoracic inoculation of *Toxorhynchites* mosquitoes (which do not take blood meals) or Aedes mosquitoes has been used. In routine diagnosis, the C6/36 cell lines have become most widely used. Following a period of 7–10 days postinoculation in cell lines or 14 days postinoculation in mosquitoes, virus identification is done by immunofluorescence assay with serotype-specific monoclonal antibodies
- *Coxiella burnetii* is an obligate intracellular organism. It is cultivated in embryonated eggs or laboratory animals like guinea pigs or mice. Seven day old embryonated chick eggs are commonly used for this purpose.
- *Rabbit ileal loop test*: A technique used to identify enterotoxins produced by *E coli* and *Salmonella spp*, in which the supernatant from these organisms in culture is inoculated into a ligated segment of ileum, which responds by 'locking' the intestinal adenylate cyclase into the 'on' position, increasing secretion of fluids into the loop of intestine.

Forensic Medicine

1. Match the following drug poisonings with their antidotes:

Drug	Antidote
1. HCN	A. Trimethadione
2. Paracetamol	B. Naloxone
3. Morphine	C. Bupropion
4. Nicotine	D. Diazepam
	E. N-acetyl cysteine
	F. Amyl nitrite

Ans. **1-F, 2-E, 3-B, 4-A**

Common Antidotes and their Indications

Antidote	Indication
Acetylcysteine	Acetaminophen
Amyl nitrite	Cyanide
Atropine sulfate	Organophosphorus and carbamate pesticides
Benztropine	Drug-induced dystonia
Bicarbonate, sodium	Na^+ channel blocking drugs
Bromocriptine	Neuroleptic malignant syndrome
Calcium gluconate or chloride	Ca^{2+} channel blocking drugs, fluoride
Carnitine	Valproate hyperammonemia
Dantrolene	Malignant hyperthermia
Deferoxamine	Iron
Digoxin immune Fab	Cardiac glycosides
Dimercaprol (BAL)	Lead, mercury, arsenic
EDTA, $CaNa_2$	Lead
Ethanol	Methanol, ethylene glycol
Fomepizole	Methanol, ethylene glycol
Flumazenil	Benzodiazepines
Glucagon hydrochloride	β adrenergic antagonists
Hydroxocobalamin hydrochloride	Cyanide
Insulin (high dose)	Ca^{2+} channel blockers

Contd…

Contd...

Antidote	Indication
Leucovorin calcium	Methotrexate
Methylene blue	Methemoglobinemia
Naloxone	Opioids
Octreotide acetate	Sulfonylurea-induced hypoglycemia
Oxygen, hyperbaric	Carbon monoxide
Penicillamine	Lead, mercury, copper
Physostigmine salicylate	Anticholinergic syndrome
Pralidoxime chloride (2-PAM)	Organophosphorus pesticides
Pyridoxine hydrochloride	Isoniazid seizures
Succimer (DMSA)	Lead, mercury, arsenic
Thiosulfate, sodium	Cyanide
Trimathadione	Nicotine
Vitamin K_1 (phytonadione)	Coumarin, indanedion

2. Which of the following types of toxins has the maximum damage potential?

a. Irritant poison
b. Corrosive poison
c. Alcohol
d. Opioid

Ans. b. Corrosive poison

Corrosive Poisoning

Poisoning by Acids

- Acids are potent desiccants and produce immediate coagulative necrosis of tissues.
  - Hydrofluoric acid (HF) is an exception, because it produces liquefactive necrosis.
- An eschar is formed at the site of exposure, which then limits further damage.
- *Mechanism of eschar formation*: When a strong acid is mixed with a solvent, large amount of heat is produced. This thermochemical reaction results in eschar formation.
- Stronger acid solutions with lower pH (higher H^+ content) are more corrosive.
- Acid causes greater damage to gastric mucosa than esophageal mucosa because squamous epithelium is more resistant to acid exposure. However, when exposed to alkali, esophageal mucosa is more severely damaged.

- Antrum and pylorus are most commonly affected parts of the stomach.
- Irritants produce less severe damage than corrosives and produces symptoms simulating gastroenteritis

3. Match the following:

1. Marsh test	A. Morphine
2. Silver nitrate paper test	B. Arsenic
3. Marquis test	C. Ethanol
4. Dichromate test	D. Hydrochloric acid

Ans. 1–B, 2–D, 3–A, 4–C

Diagnostic tests used for poisoning by various agents are enlisted below:

Trinder's test	Aspirin
FPN test	Phenothiazines
O-cresol test	Paracetamol
Fujiwara test	Chloral hydrate, chloroform
Dithionate test	Paraquat
Dichromate test	Ethanol
Reinsch test, Marsh test	Arsenic
Marquis test	Morphine
Meixner test	Mushroom poisoning
Silver nitrate test	Hydrochloric acid

4. Which of the following is/are toxins?

1. All are correct	A. Atropine
2. a, b, c correct	B. Colchicine
3. a and c correct	C. Curare
4. c and d are correct	D. Arsenic

Ans. 1. All are correct

All of the given agents can act as toxins.

Toxins are classified as follows:

Corrosive poisons:

- *Inorganic or mineral acids*: Sulphuric acid, Nitric acid
- *Organic acids*: Carbolic acid, Oxalic acid, Hydrochloric acid
- *Alkalis*: Carbonates and hydroxides of sodium and potassium
- Irritant poisons
- *Inorganic*: Nonmetallic—Phosphorus, Halogens; Metallic—Arsenic, Mercury, Lead, Copper
- *Organic*: Abrus, Castor, Croton, Calotropis, Ergot
- Systemic poisons
- CNS:
    - *Somniferous*: Opium, pethidine
    - *Inebriants*: Alcohol, anesthetics, sedative hypnotics, insecticides, hydrocarbons, Benzodiazepines
    - *Delirients*: Dhatura, cannabis, cocaine

- *Spinal*: Strychnine, gelsemium
- *Peripheral*: Curare, conium
- *CVS*: Oleander, aconite, nicotine
- *Ashpyxiants*: CO, CO_2, cyanogen gas, cyanides

5. Identify the postmortem change depicted in the given image:

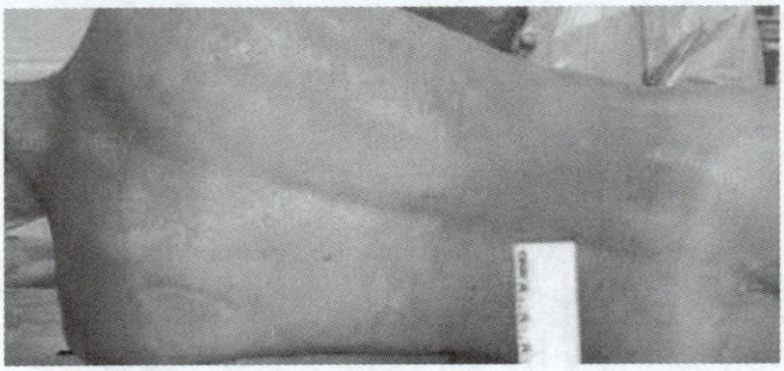

a. Pallor mortis
b. Algor mortis
c. Postmortem hypostasis
d. Postmortem marbling

Ans. c. Postmortem hypostasis

- Livor mortis, also known as hypostasis, is the discoloration of the skin due to the pooling of blood in the dependent parts of the body following death. The blood pools because the heart can no longer circulate the blood. Gravity will make the blood settle and the areas where it settles turns to a dark blue or purple color, which is termed 'lividity'.
- The blood begins to pool immediately following death and is visible within a couple of hours. After the first two hours, the skin is bluish and blotchy. After five or six hours, the blotches become confluent and the skin will turn white when applied with pressure. After ten to twelve hours, the livid color remains even when pressed.
- It is important to note that the blood will migrate to the lowest point in the body that it can travel. This may not necessarily be the lowest part of the body. For instance, if the victim was a hanging victim, the lividity will show in the feet, fingertips and earlobes. If the body is found in a supine position, the lividity will be found in the parts of the body touching the ground. Being able to identify the discoloration can be very useful in determining if a body has been moved after death.

6. Mark whether the following clauses of 320 IPC are true/false with respect to their sequence:

a. Second→ Permanent privation of the sight of either eye
b. First→ Emasculation
c. Eight→ Fracture or dislocation of a bone or tooth
d. Sixth→ Permanent disfiguration of the head or face
e. None

Ans. a–T, b–T, c–F, d–T

Sec–320 IPC– Grievous hurt—the following kinds of hurt only are designated as "grievous":

1. *Firstly*: Emasculation
2. *Secondly*: Permanent privation of the sight of either eye.
3. *Thirdly*: Permanent privation of the hearing of either ear.
4. *Fourthly*: Privation of any member or joint.
5. *Fifthly*: Destruction or permanent impairing of the powers of any member or joint.
6. *Sixthly*: Permanent disfiguration of the head or face.
7. *Seventhly*: Fracture or dislocation of a bone or tooth.
8. *Eighthly*: Any hurt which endangers life or which causes the sufferer to be during the space of twenty days in severe bodily pain, or unable to follow his ordinary pursuits

7. What is the most likely cause of injury shown in the given image? (In the image given, right eye ball was missing, with lacerations in the periorbital area and hematoma within the bony orbit)?

a. Blunt rupture to eyeball
b. Evisceration by sharp weapon
c. Post mortem artefact
d. None of the Above

Ans. b. Evisceration by sharp weapon

- Missing eyeball in a dead body indicates either antemortem evisceration or removal of the eyeball postmortem. If the eyeball was removed after the death of the individual, no hematoma would have been formed. Hematoma within the orbit indicates antemortem injury. Lacerations in the adjacent skin also suggest injury by a sharp weapon.
- In blunt rupture of eye, the complete eye will not be missing. Following are the types of ocular injuries associated with blunt trauma.

Eyelids	Ecchymosis, swelling, laceration, abrasions, conjunctival, or subconjunctival hemorrhages
Cornea	Edema, lacerations
Anterior chamber	Hyphema, recession of angle, secondary glaucoma
Iris	Iridodialysis, iridoplegia, rupture of iris sphincter
Ciliary body	Hyposecretion of aqueous humor
Lens	Cataract, dislocation
Vitreous	Vitreous hemorrhage
Ciliary muscle	Paralysis
Retina	Commotio retinae, retinal edema, choroidal breaks in Bruch membrane, choroidal hemorrhage

8. What is the appropriate management of the injury given in the image?

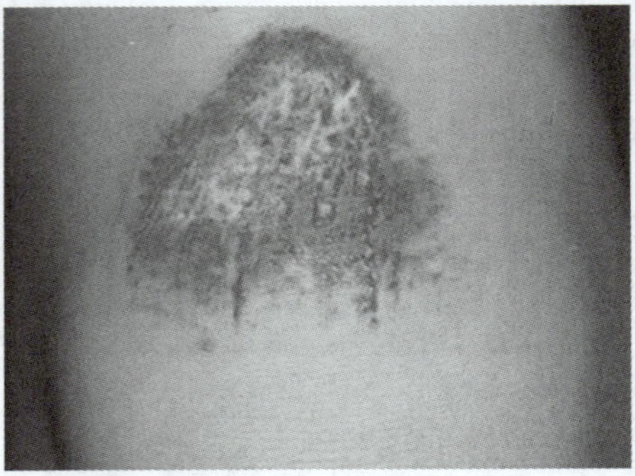

a. Debridement and dressing
b. Cleaning and dressing
c. Dressing
d. Suture and dressing

Ans. b. Cleaning and dressing

Abrasion: Also called gravel rash, is the destruction of the superficial layer of the epidermis.

Features

1. Caused by friction against a rough surface or by compression
2. Simple injury which heals rapidly without scar formation. The exception is corneal abrasion which is a grievous injury.
3. Bleed less

Types

1. Scratch e.g. nail marks, abrasion by pin, thorn
2. *Graze*: Most common type. Characterised by uneven, longitudinal parallel grooves and furrows with heaped of epithelium at one end, which indicate direction of force.
3. Pressure, e.g. bite marks, ligature marks over neck in hanging and strangulation.
4. *Imprint*: Reflect the pattern of object which produces the abrasion, e.g. tyre marks in RTA.

Most abrasions can be managed by cleaning the wound using an antiseptic solution followed by dressing. Debridement is done for infected wounds. Suture is not necessary as there is no discontinuity in the skin.

9. Assertion/Reason

Assertion: The range from which a shotgun was fired can be determined by examining the dispersion of pellets

Reason: Multiple pellets are present in shotgun

a. Both Assertion and Reasoning are independently true/correct and Reason is the correct explanation of the Assertion
b. Both Assertion and Reasoning are independently true/correct and Reason is not the correct explanation of the Assertion
c. Assertion is independently a true/correct statement but the Reason is independently an incorrect/false statement
d. Assertion is independently a false/incorrect statement but the Reason is independently a true/correct statement
e. Both Assertion and Reason are independently a false/incorrect statement

Ans. a. Both Assertion and Reasoning are independently true/correct and Reason is the correct explanation of the Assertion

Characteristics of shotgun wound at various ranges are given below:

Characteristics	Range/distance of firing						
	Contact shot	***Close shot ranges***			***Near shot***	***Distant shot***	
Range	Contact range	Close range	Short to Mid range			Mid to distant range	
	In touch	<15 cm	15 cm	90 cm	2 m	4 m	20 m
Number of wounds	Single	Single	Single	Single	Multiple	Multiple	Multiple
Spread area	–	–	–	–	5–7 cm	10–14 cm	>14 cm
Site	Vital parts	Any where on the body					
Size	Largest (>2.5 cm)	Smaller	Smallest	Rat hole	Central big wound with smaller wounds around	Wider spread	Spread is not measurable
Edges	Scorched and contused	Well defined and inverted		Irregular and lacerated	–	–	–
Blackening	+++	+++	++	+	–	–	–
Tattooing	+++	++++	+++	++	–	–	–
Singeing	+++	++++	++	–	–	–	–

Contd..

10. Paradoxical undressing seen in:

a. Immersion syndrome
b. Heat cramps
c. Hypothermia
d. Heat exhaustion

Ans. c. Hypothermia

Paradoxical Undressing

It is seen in hypothermia when the victim often exhibits altered states of judgement, which is known in mountaineering circles as being "cold stupid".

Pathophysiology

As the body becomes colder, it shunts blood away from the extremities and into the warm core in order to protect vital organs. Shunting of blood to the core and away from extremities is accomplished through vasoconstriction of peripheral circulation. Vasoconstriction requires a steady input of energy in the form of glucose from the body's energy stores. However, due to a lack of blood now travelling to these muscles, they eventually exhaust. As the muscles of the constricted blood vessels run out of energy, vasodilatation occurs. With vasodilatation, an infusion of warm blood from the core of the body rushes into the peripheral extremities. This causes the hypothermia victim to feel overly warm and to start shedding layers of clothing, contrary to the reality that their body temperature is continuing to drop. The victim's warm blood rushing from their core, coupled with the removal of warm clothing, causes their body temperature to fall even faster. This serves to hasten death from hypothermia and is called paradoxical undressing.

Orthopedics

1. True/false in view of septic arthritis:

a. Widening of joint space is there
b. *Staph aureus* is the most common organism in young children and neonate
c. Incision and drainage is frequently required
d. Kocher criteria used to differentiate from transient synovitis
e. Position of hip is flexion, adduction and internal rotation

Ans. a- T, b-T, c- T, d- T, e-F

Septic (Pyogenic) Arthritis

Refers to Infection of Joint: Septic arthritis word is a misnomer as initially there is only infection of joint and if not treated early then Arthritis (joint destruction) develops. Thus, all sepsis of joints do not cause arthritis only inadequately treated ones do.

Etiology and Pathology

- The hematogenous route of infection is the most common route in all age groups.

Epidemiology

- *S. aureus*–is the most common organism.
  (Absent movements of a joint after ruling out trauma in pediatric population is septic arthritis till proved otherwise).

Order of investigations in any inflammatory joint swelling
↓
X-ray
↓
MRI
↓
Aspiration

X-ray
MRI
Aspiration
Swelling of a joint

X-M A S

Diagnosis: X-rays are usually normal or may indicate soft tissue swellings, MRI may show effusion, synovitis or cartilage destruction and aspiration of joint will help to confirm the diagnosis by culture and sensitivity and can also help to differentiate from transient synovitis. Aspiration also decreases intra-articular pressure and reduces chances of avascular necrosis (AVN) of femoral head.

- Aspiration shows > 50,000 cells/mL and >75% polymorphoneutrophils in septic arthritis.
- Culture of the aspirate is the gold standard for diagnosis.
- Kocher criterion.

Septic Arthritis with Negative Cultures–Diagnostic Criterion (Morrey and Associates Criterion)

5 out of 6 must be present

1. >38.3°C temperature
2. Swelling of suspected joint
3. Pain in joint that increases with movement
4. Systemic symptoms
5. No other pathologic process
6. Satisfactory response to antibiotics therapy.

Clinically

1. Knee (most commonly affected joint)–Position is flexion
2. Hip—Position is flexion, abduction and external rotation as this is the position of maximum capacity of joint to accommodate pus.

Treatment

Arthrotomy (opening the joint capsule), surgical drainage (decompression) synovectomy and antibiotics. (2 weeks IV and 4 weeks oral). Duration of antibiotics is same as osteomyelitis as usually focus is from the bone.

Kocher Criterion

- Non-weight-bearing on affected side
- Erythrocyte sedimentation rate > 40
- Fever > 38.5°C
- White blood cell count >12,000

2. True/False about fracture shaft of femur:

a. More commonly in elderly
b. Easily managed with gallows traction in elderly
c. Associated with pulmonary complications
d. Intramedullary nailing is gold standard for management

Ans. a-F, b-F, c-T, d-T

Fracture Shaft Femur–Age-wise Treatment

- *<5 years*: Spica
- *≥5 years*: Nailing
- *5–10 years*: Close reduction and internal fixation with Elastic Nails (TENS)
- *≥ 10 years*: Closed interlock nailing.

Fracture Femur with Breathlessness after 48 hours think of it!

Fat embolism refers to the presence of fat globules in vital organs and peripheral circulation after fracture of a long bone or other major trauma. Fat embolism syndrome reflects a serious systemic manifestation as a consequence to these emboli.

- Fat embolism is a common phenomenon. It is more commonly seen in patients with multiple fractures and in fractures involving lower limbs especially femur.
- Fat originates from the site of trauma, particularly from the injured marrow. Fat globules > 10 mm are considered significant.

Clinical Presentation

- Early warning signs are a slight rise in temperature and pulse rate (tachycardia)
  The classical triad of fat embolism syndrome is:
  1. *Respiratory symptoms*: Dyspnea or tachypnea.
  2. *Neurological symptoms*: Confusion or disorientation.
  3. *Petechial rash*: In axilla, neck, periumbilical area, conjunctiva of lower lid, front and back of chest, shoulder.
- Fat embolism is rare in children.

Diagnostic Criterion for Fat Embolism

Gurd's Major Criteria (4)

Axillary or subconjunctival petechia

- PaO_2 below 60 mm Hg
- CNS depression
- Pulmonary edema

Gurd's Minor Criteria (8)

- Tachycardia
- Fever
- Anemia
- Thrombocytopenia
- Fat globules in sputum
- Fat globules in urine (Gurd test)
- Increasing ESR

- Retinal emboli
- 1 major + 4 minor = fat embolism

Prevention

1. Fracture stabilization
2. Removing fat emboli from circulation by:
   a. Lipolytic agents as heparin (increase serum lipase activity)
   b. Hypertonic glucose (decrease FFA production)
3. Offset its effect by:
   a. Dextran (expand plasma volume, reduces RBC aggregation and platelet adherence)
   b. Aprotinin (protease inhibitor) decreases platelet aggregation and serotonin release.
   c. Alcohol has vasodilator and lipolytic effect.

Treatment

The aim of treatment is maintaining adequate oxygen level in the blood. If necessary by using intermittent positive pressure ventilation. Oxygen is the only therapeutic tool of proven use. It should be administered in sufficient amount to maintain arterial PO_2 > 80 mm Hg. O_2 toxicity (pneumonitis) is avoided by using O_2 conc. below 40%.
Steroids are given to avoid pneumonitis.

Waddell's triad: Head injury; Fracture shaft femur and intraabdominal/ intrathoracic injury.

3. Most specific for diagnosing ankylosing spondylitis:

a. HLA B27
b. Bilateral sacroilitis
c. Lumbar movements
d. ESR

Ans. b. Bilateral sacroilitis

Ankylosing Spondylitis

Diagnostic Criteria–Modified New York Criterion

- Essential criteria is definite radiographic Sacroiliitis
- Supporting criteria: one of these three

Inflammatory Back Pain

- Limited chest expansion (<5 cm at 4th ICS) {not a reliable criterion in elderly because of pulmonary disorders}
- Limited lumbar spine motion in both sagittal and frontal plane (Schober test/Modified Schober test).
- Inflammatory back pain is classified if 4/5 are present
  1. Pain for > 3 months

2. <40 years age
3. Insidious onset
4. Pain improves with exercise
5. Pain at night

Sacroiliitis

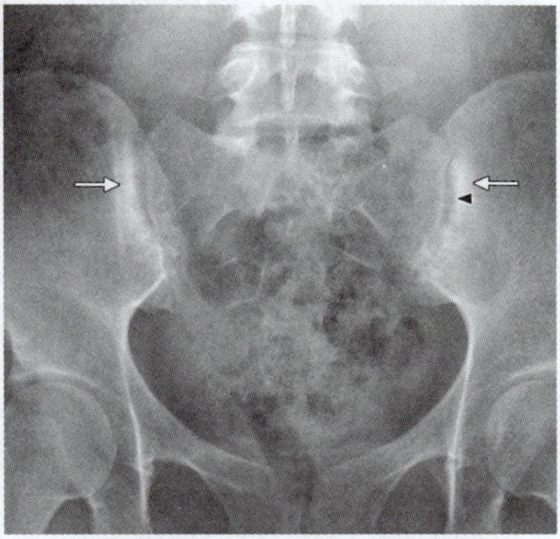

AS (Ankylosing spondilitis)

- Bamboo spine
- Squaring of vertebra

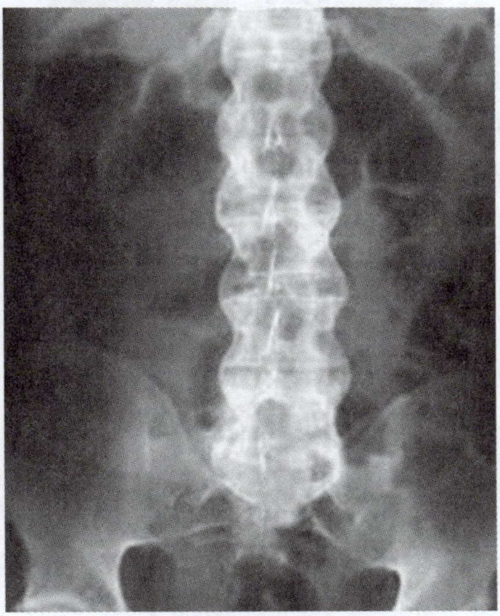

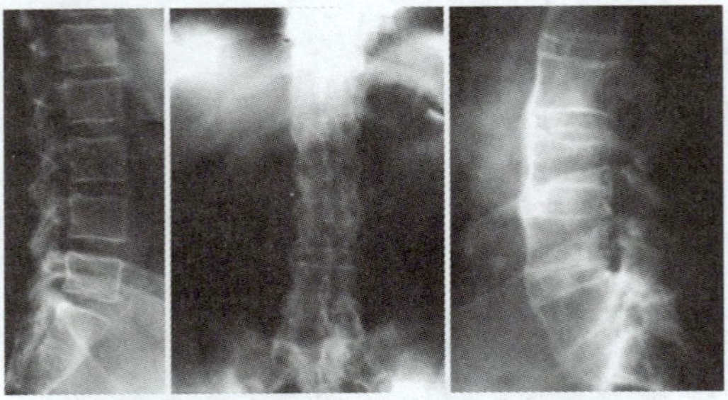

Dagger Sign

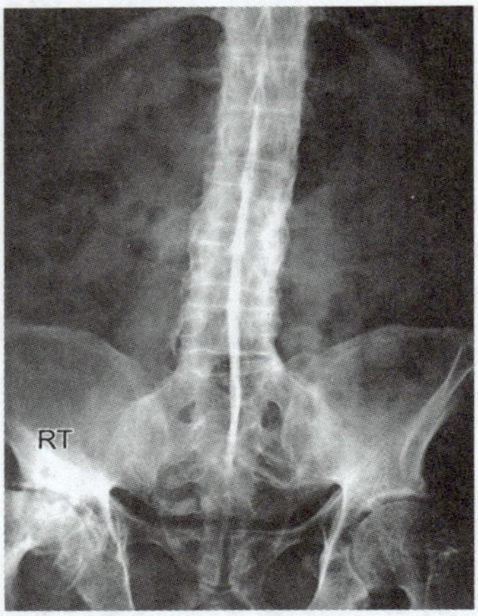

Trolley Track Sign

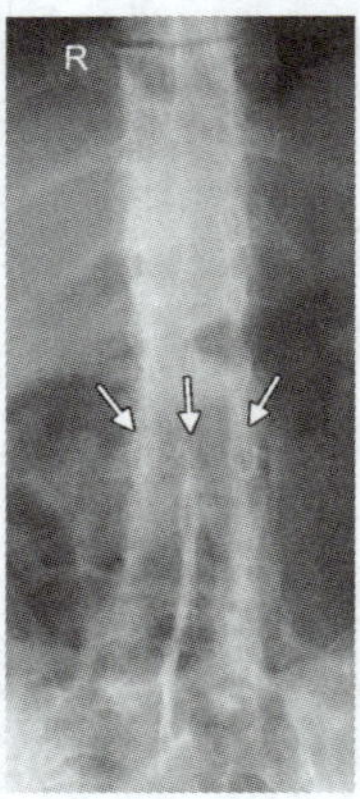

Romanus Sign

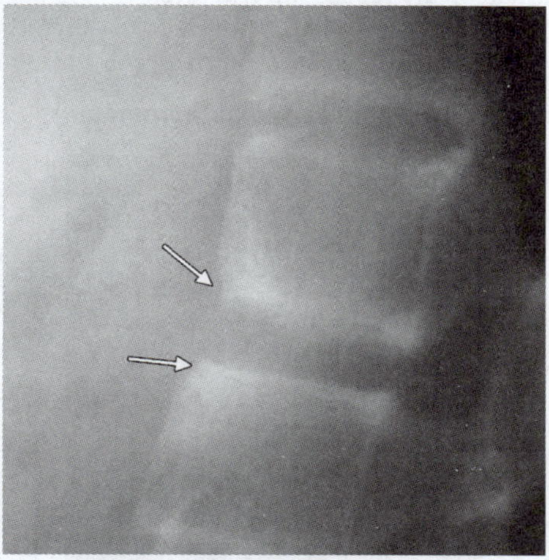

4. A 75-year-female had a fall and had intertrochanteric fracture. This is due to:

a. Osteoporosis b. Osteopetrosis
c. Paget's disease d. Metastasis

Ans. a. Osteoporosis

Comparison of osteoporosis and osteomalacia

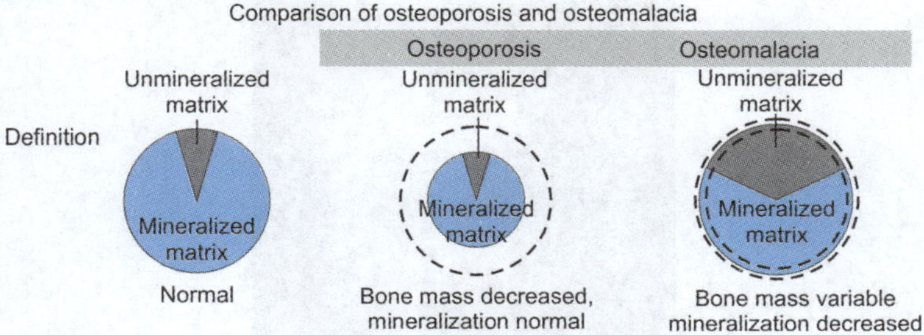

Osteoporosis (V>H>C)

- Bone mineral density—DEXA scan …65 years onwards
- T score
- 0 to –1–Normal
- –1 to –2.5–Osteopenia
- <–2.5 –Osteoporosis
- Severe osteoporosis?
- Normal Ca, PO_4, Alp
- Hemiplegic-Humerus maximum loss of bone mineral density

- Estrogen
- Bisphosphonates—Increases hip fracture
- Calcitonin
- Low dose PTH—stimulates osteoblasts

Codfish Vertebrae (Osteoporosis/Osteomalacia)

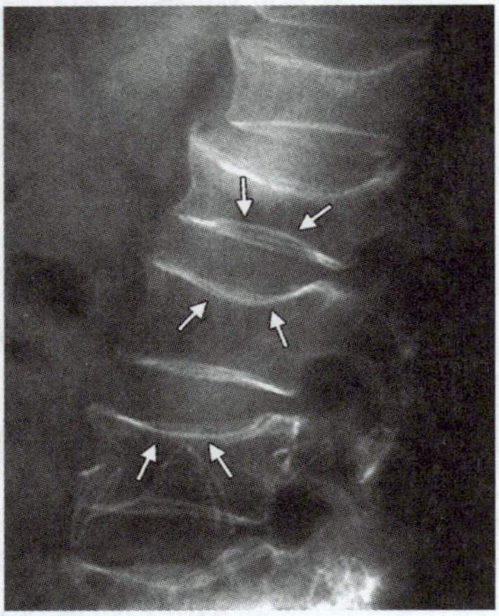

5. What to be done next?

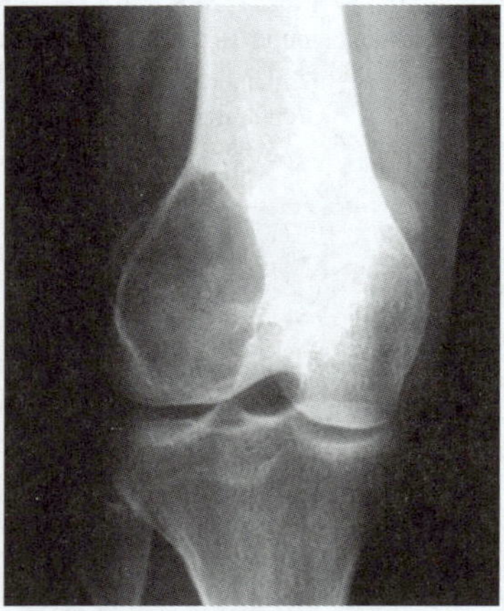

a. Extended curettage with allograft
b. Bone biopsy
c. Curettage
d. Extended curettage with autograft

Ans. b. Bone biopsy

They typically occur in patients 20–40 years old, and there is a slight female predominance. The most common location for this tumor is the distal femur, followed closely by the proximal tibia.

Tumor of lower end radius is GCT till proved otherwise.

Multiple giant cell like bone tumors—Goltz syndrome. GCT has egg shell crackling on palpation.

Although these tumors typically are benign, pulmonary metastases occur in approximately 3% of patients.

Malignant giant cell tumors represent less than 5% of total GCT. Malignancy in GCT-Osteosarcoma or Malignant Fibrous Histiocytoma or Fibrosarcoma.

Radiographic findings often are diagnostic. The lesions are eccentrically located in the epiphyses of long bones and usually about the subchondral bone. Although rare in skeletally immature patients, giant cell tumors arise in the metaphysis in this age group.

Radiographically, the lesions are purely lytic. The lesion frequently expands or breaks through the cortex; however, intraarticular extension is rare because the subchondral bone usually remains intact.

Microscopically, giant cell tumors are composed of many multinucleated giant cells (typically 40–60 nuclei per cell) in a sea of mononuclear stromal cells (malignant cells). The nuclei of the mononuclear cells are identical to the nuclei of the giant cells, a feature that helps to distinguish giant cell tumors from other tumors that may contain many giant cells.

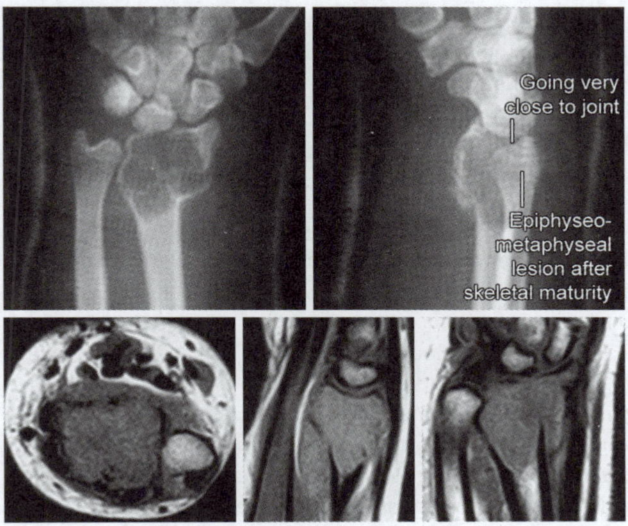

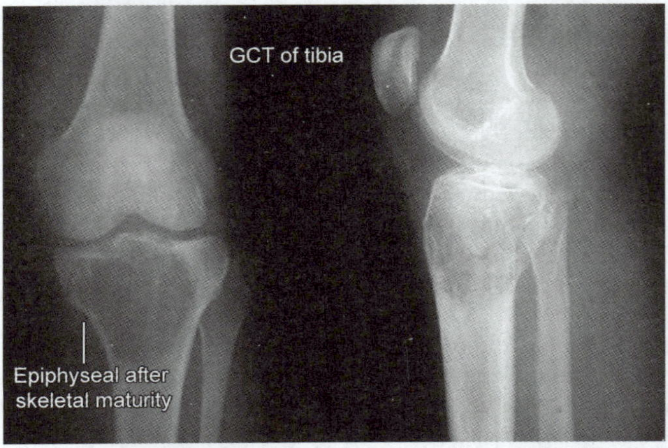

Giant cell tumor of lower end radius (F). Giant cell tumor of upper end tibia.

Giant Cell Variants (Tumor with Giant Cells)

- Brown tumor of hyperparathyroidism
- Aneurysmal bone cyst (closest) and unicameral bone cyst
- Non-ossifying fibroma (commonest) and Fibrous dysplasia
- Osteoblastoma and osteosarcoma
- Metastatic carcinoma with giant cells
- Chondromyxoid fibroma and chondroblastoma
- Pigmented villonodular synovitis (mostly occurring in knee)
- Benign fibrous histiocytoma
- Malignant fibrous histiocytoma
- Fibrosarcoma
- Clear cell chondrosarcoma.

Treatment of Osteoclastoma (GCT)

1. Extended curettage by PMMA or phenol or liquid nitrogen and bone grafting. It is procedure of choice for most lesions.
2. Excision
   - Lower end of ulna
   - Upper end of fibula
3. Excision and replacement by vascularized bone graft. Lower end of radius where upper end of fibula is grafted
4. Excision and arthrodesis or prosthetic replacement or Turn:
   - O–Plasty (Bone ends are cut and rotated)
   - Lower end femur and upper end tibia

5. Treatment of recurrent lesions is the same as for primary lesions. After biopsy shows that the tumor is still benign, repeat curettage or resection should be performed.
6. *Amputation*: Malignant recurrent GCT of extremity
7. *Radiotherapy*: Spine (RT may cause malignant transformation of GCT).

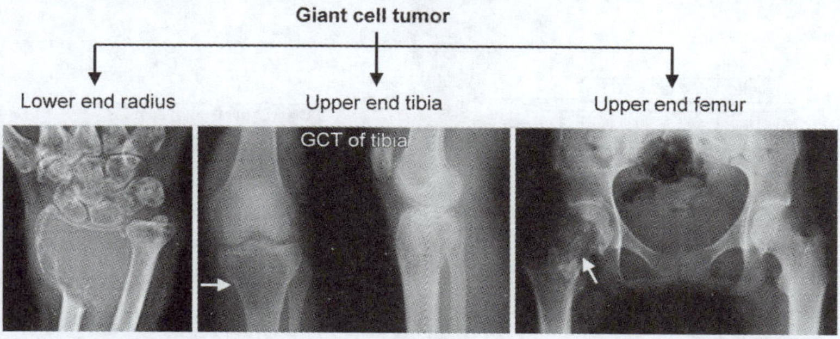

Lower End Femur

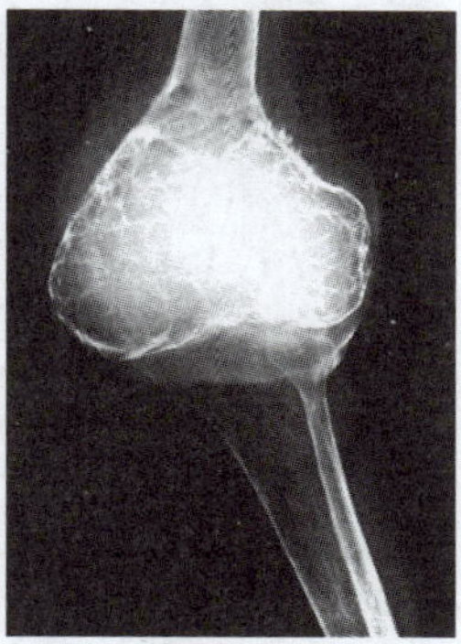

6. Match the Eponym with their fractures:

Eponym	Fracture
1. Pilon's fracture	a. Trimalleolar ankle fracture (medial, lateral and posterior malleolar) fracture
2. Runners fracture	b. Comminuted depressed fracture of the lateral tibial condyle
3. Cotton's fracture	c. Comminuted intra-articular fracture of distal tibial end
4. Chauffer's fracture	d. Fracture lower end fibula

e. An intra-articular oblique fracture of the styloid process of the radius.

f. Bimalleolar ankle fracture

Ans. **1-c, 2-d, 3-a, 4-e**

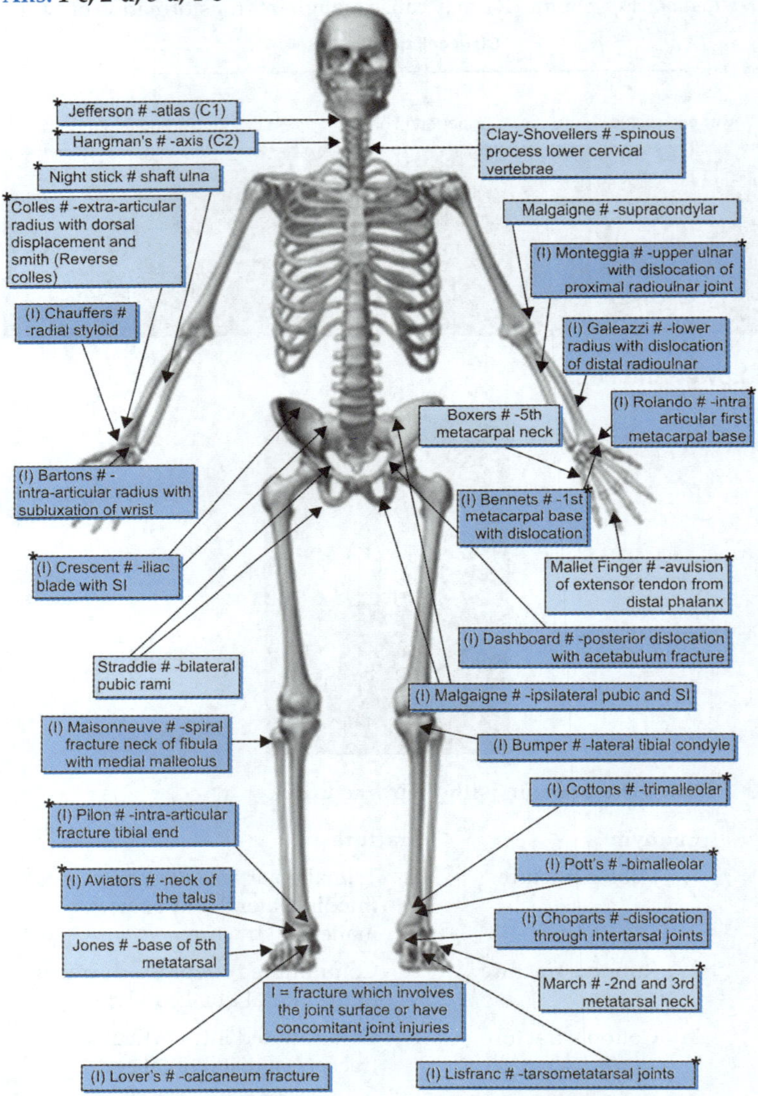

***Latest Questions**

Night Stick Fracture

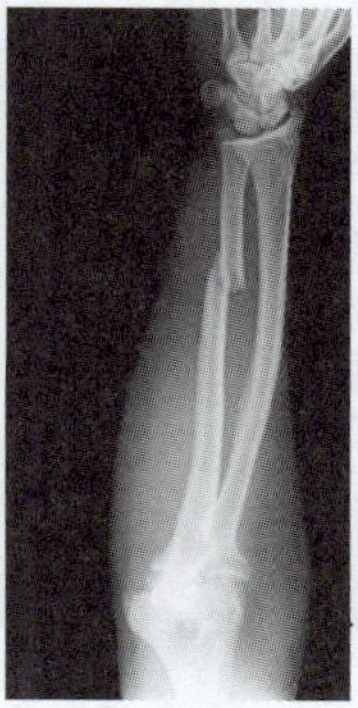

Chauffeur Fracture

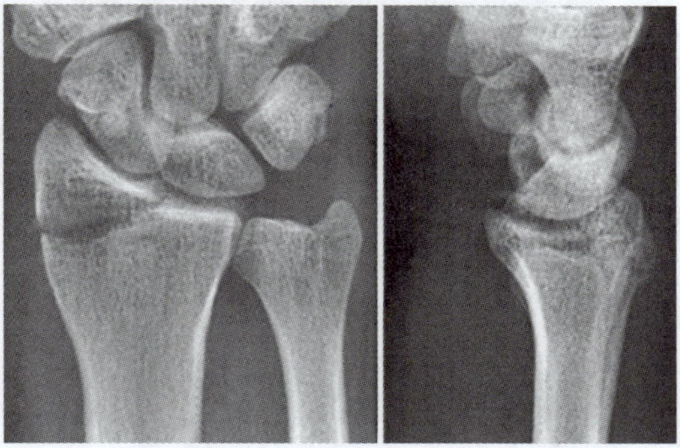

Bumper Fracture

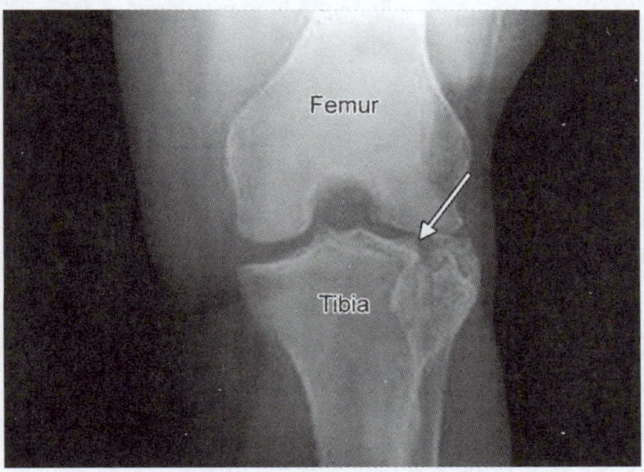

Pott's Fracture

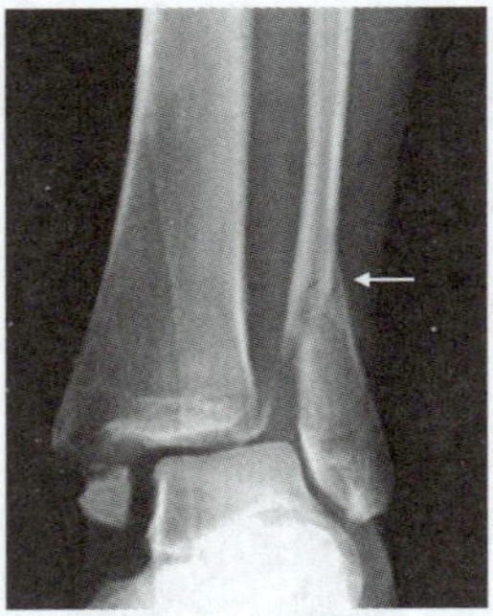

Cotton Fracture

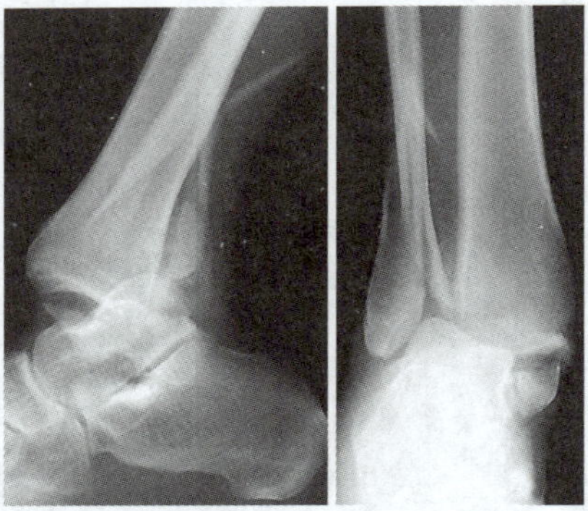

Runner Fracture

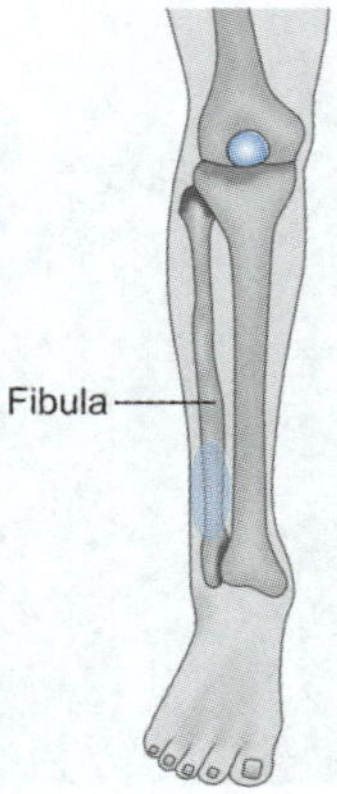

7. The instrument shown in the image is used for:

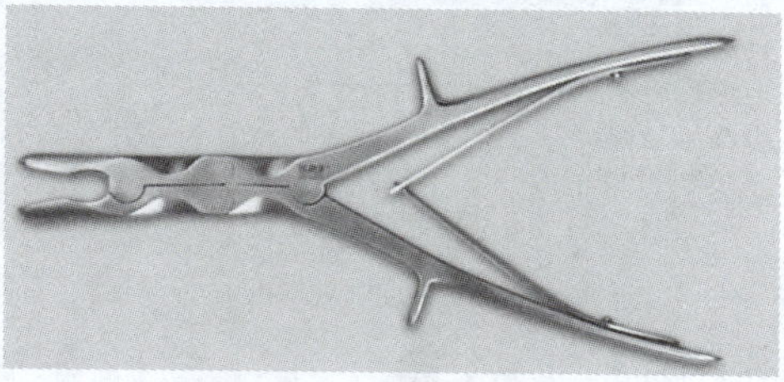

a. For cutting ribs in thoracic surgery
b. For smoothening of edges in amputation surgery
c. Used as a bone nibbler
d. To remove fibrous tissue from non-union site

Ans. c. Used as a bone nibbler

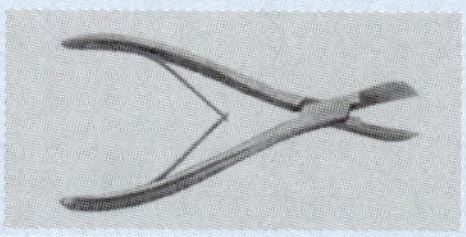 Bone Cutter	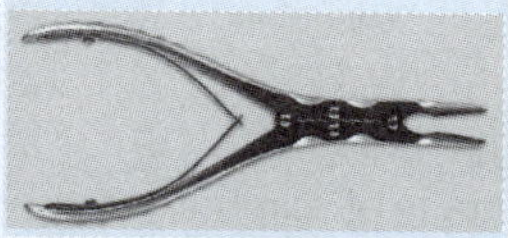 Bone Nibbler Double Action	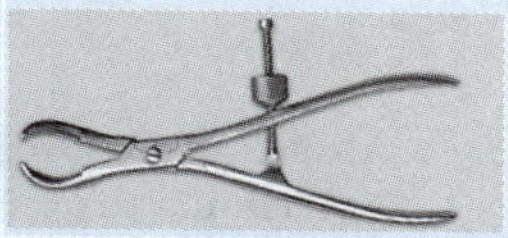 Bone Holding Forceps
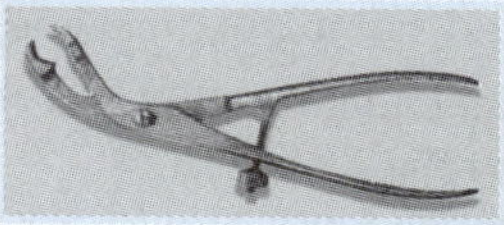 Bone Plate Holding Forceps	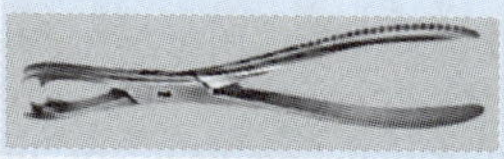 Fergusson Bone Holding Forceps	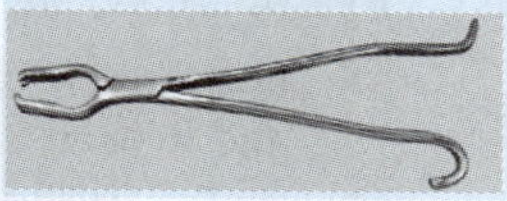 Lane Bone Holding Forceps
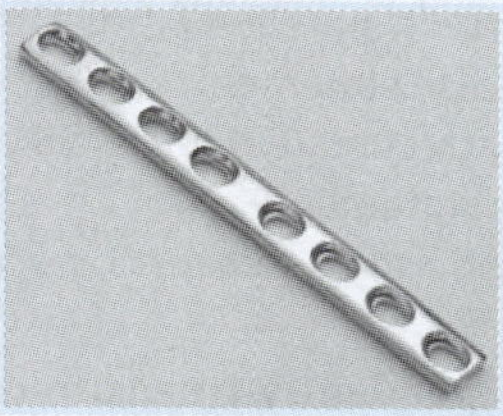 Dynamic Compression Plate (DCP)	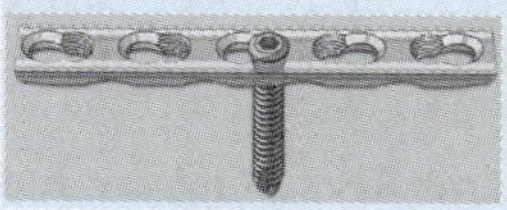 Locking Compression Plate (LCP)	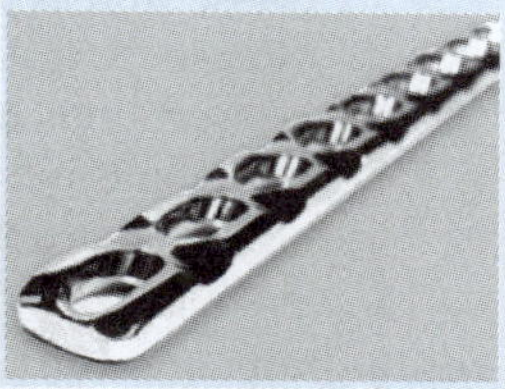 Limited Contact Dynamic Compression Plate (LCDCP)
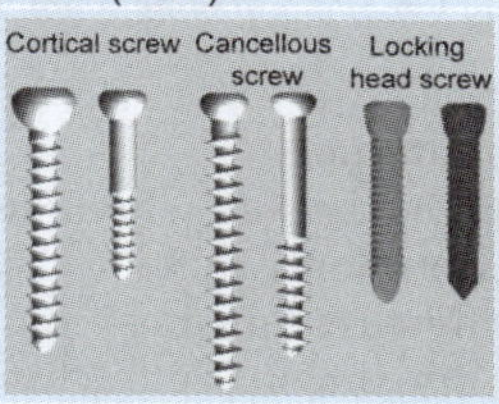 Screws	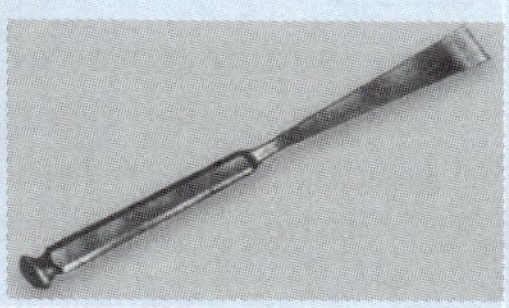 Osteotome	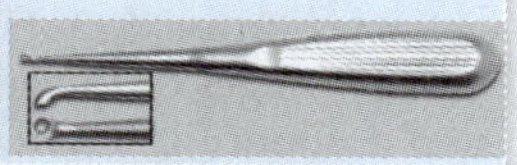 Bone Curette

Contd...

Contd...

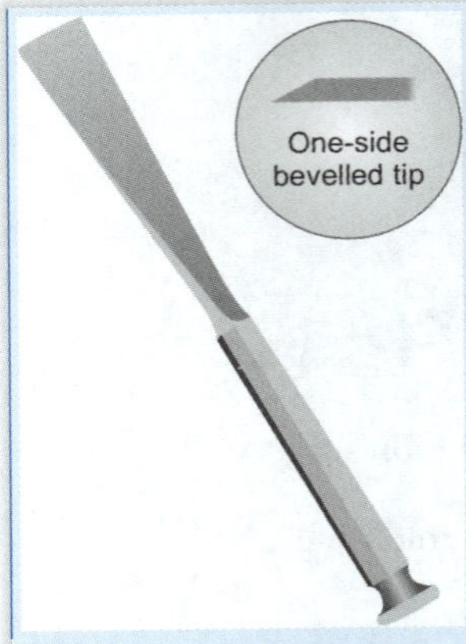

Chisel

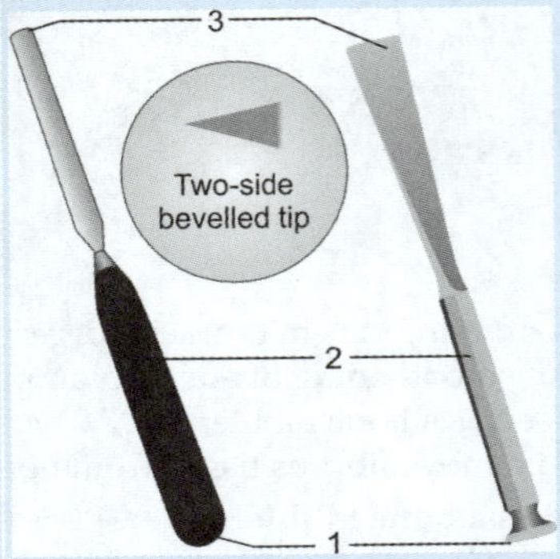

Osteotome

8. Assertion reason:

Assertion: Proximal pole of scaphoid is the most common bone to undergo avascular necrosis

Reason: Blood supply is retrograde from its distal to proximal end

a. Both Assertion and Reasoning are independently true/correct and Reason is the correct explanation of the Assertion

b. Both Assertion and Reasoning are independently true/correct and Reason is not the correct explanation of the Assertion

c. Assertion is independently a true/correct statement but the Reason is independently an incorrect/false statement

d. Assertion is independently a false/incorrect statement but the Reason is independently a true/correct statement

e. Both Assertion and Reason are independently a false/incorrect statement

Ans. a. Both Assertion and Reasoning are independently true/correct and Reason is the correct explanation of the Assertion

Relative Incidence of Carpal Bone Fractures

Scaphoid > Triquetral >Trapezium

Fracture Scaphoid—Tenderness in anatomical snuff box!

Scaphoid is the most commonly fractured bone in the carpus, in adult as well as children. Scaphoid fracture is seen most commonly in males between the ages of 15 and 30. Middle third (Waist) fractures are most common accounting for 70% of scaphoid fractures > proximal pole fracture (20%) > distal pole fracture (10%), in adults and adolescents. Distal pole avulsion type fracture is most common fracture type in children.

- Most of the blood supply to the scaphoid enters distally, so blood supply of scaphoid diminishes proximally. This accounts for the fact that 1% of distal third, 20% of middle third, 40% of proximal third and 100% of proximal pole fractures result in avascular necrosis or non-union of the proximal fragment.

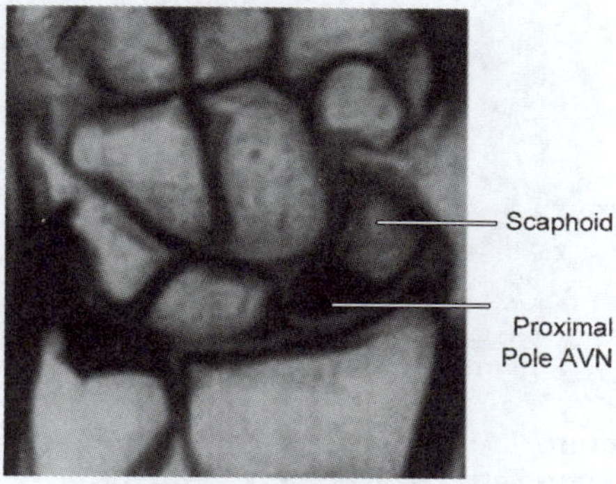

AVN scaphoid

- A delay in diagnosis and treatment of this fracture may alter the prognosis for union.
- A wrist sprain that is sufficiently severe to require radiographic examination initially should be treated as a possible fracture of the scaphoid, and radiographs should be repeated in 2 weeks even though initial radiographs may be negative.
- Fullness and tenderness in anatomical snuff box. Proximal pressure along the axis of the thumb may be painful.
- Recent fracture shows only in the oblique view.
- MRI can diagnose occult fractures.
- MRI, especially with gadolinium enhancement, also is useful in assessing the vascularity of a fractured scaphoid.

Nondisplaced, Stable Scaphoid Fractures: Scaphoid Glass Holding Cast

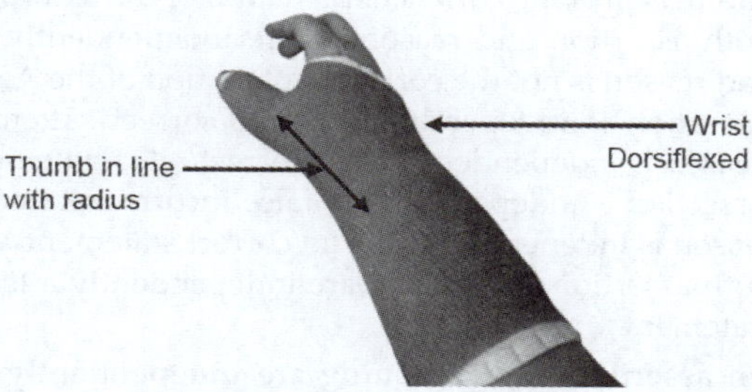

Glass holding cast—scaphoid

Displaced, unstable scaphoid fractures: Headless screw (Herbert) is used

- Complication nonunion > avascular necrosis.

Blood Supply Distal to Proximal

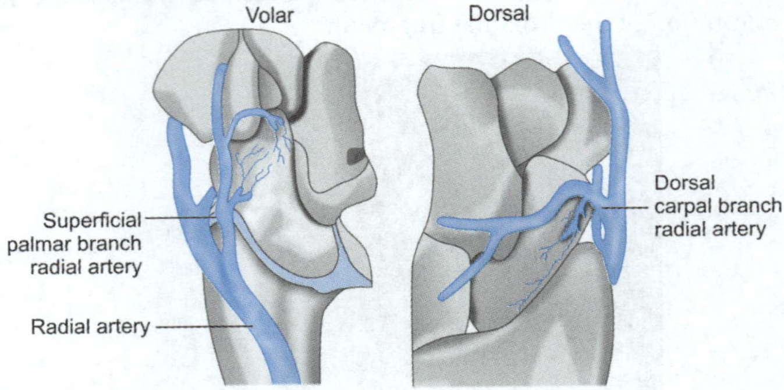

Scaphoid Fracture

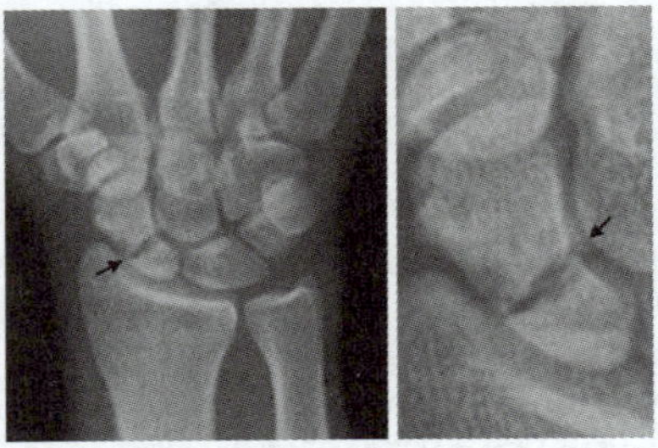

9. Assertion Reason:

Assertion: Decompression surgery is needed with progressive neurological difficulty in Pott's spine.

Reason: Even after completion of ATT there can be neurological abnormalities.

a. Both assertion and reasoning are independently true/correct and reason is the correct explanation of the assertion
b. Both assertion and reasoning are independently true/correct and reason is not the correct explanation of the Assertion
c. Assertion is independently a true/correct statement but the Reason is independently an incorrect/false statement
d. Assertion is independently a false/incorrect statement but the reason is independently a true/correct statement
e. Both assertion and reason are independently a false/incorrect statement

Ans. **b. Both assertion and reasoning are independently true/correct and reason is not the correct explanation of the Assertion**

Treatment of Pott's Spine

- Middle path regimen is used in India
- Patient is treated by antitubercular therapy (ATT), spinal brace and rest. Patient is followed on with complete neural examination and if progress is good then continued on nonoperative management but if indications of surgery exist then he needs to be operated.

Stage-wise Treatment of Pott's Spine

- Stage 1: ATT + rest + monthly neural examination
- Stage 2: ATT + rest + weekly neural examination
- Stage 3: ATT + rest + daily neural examination
- Stage 4: ATT + Decompression and bone grafting

ATT: Rifampicin is always a part of all regimens. Minimum duration is 9–12 months in spinal TB and may be given up to 18–24 months depending upon clinical, radiological (MRI) and hematological (ESR) healing (in non-spinal TB the duration of ATT is 6 months–1 year).

Indications of surgery in any disease of spine (These are for all pathologies of spine—trauma, tumor, TB, disk prolapse)

- Bowel bladder involvement.
- Deterioration in neural or clinical status on treatment
- No improvement in neural or clinical status after conservative trial of 3–4 weeks or

Surgical options for most of the cases are—anterior decompression + bone grafting or anterolateral decompression + bone grafting and both have similar success rates.

- Hong Kong operation is also carried out for Pott's spine.

Structures removed in anterolateral decompression are part of rib, one side transverse process, one pedicle and small part of vertebral body (intercostal nerves are exposed).

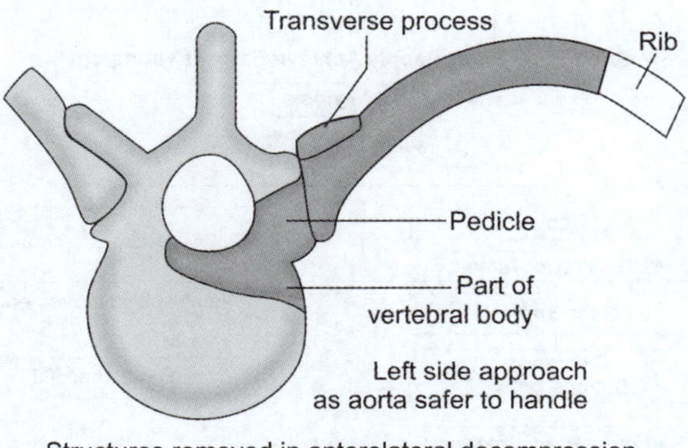

Structures removed in anterolateral decompression.

Posterior structures like lamina are never removed in tuberculosis because disease destroys anteriorly and if surgeon destroys posteriorly then there will be instability.

These surgeries are carried out in right lateral position (right side down and left side up) approaching the spine from left side as the vessel handled is aorta on left side which is thick muscular vessel with more resilience to handling pressure as compared to vena cava on right side which is friable to handle.

Prognostic Factors

Feature	Better prognosis	Poor prognosis
Degree of cord involvement	Partial	Complete (grade IV)
Duration of cord involvement	Shorter	Longer (>12 months)
Speed onset	Slow	Rapid
Type	Early onset	Late onset
Age	Younger	Older
General condition	Good	Poor
Vertebral disease	Active	Healed
Kyphotic deformity	<60°	>60°
Cord on MRI	Normal	Myelomalacia/syrinx (cord damaged)
Preoperative	Wet lesion	Dry lesion

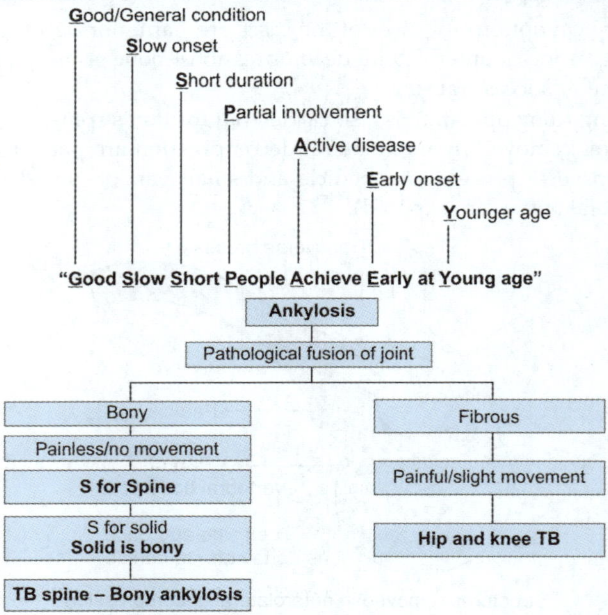

Immunomodulation

In case response to ATT is not on the expected ground and it is suspected that patient's immune system is not controlling the disease then immunomodulation is done to enhance the immune response. In immunomodulation the following sets of bacilli are attacked—dormant/resistant/persistent/slow grower/atypical m TB.

Drugs given are:

1. Levamisole
2. BCG
3. DPT

- Treatment ATT + Rest + Surgery when indicated.
- Indications of surgery in any disease of spine:
  Bowel bladder involvement
  Worsening.
  No improvement.

Ophthalmology

1. When should a patient with type 2 diabetes for one year with no other complications should have an ophthalmic examination?

a. As early as possible
b. After 5 years
c. After 10 years
d. Only after vision loss sets in

Ans. a. As early as possible

Screening for Diabetic Retinopathy

Early detection and timely treatment of diabetic retinopathy are essential for prevention of permanent visual loss. Screening should be performed within 3 years from diagnosis in type 1 diabetes, at diagnosis in type 2 diabetes, and annually thereafter in both types. Diabetic retinopathy may progress rapidly during pregnancy, and screening should take place in the first trimester and then at least every 3 months until delivery. Digital fundal photography is an effective and sensitive screening method. Seven-field photography after pupil dilation has been the gold standard, but using two 45° fields, one centered on the macula and the other centered on the disk, has been the method of choice in most screening programs.

2. A patient comes to the trauma centre with an injury as shown in the image. Which of the following steps should not be done during the initial evaluation of the patient?

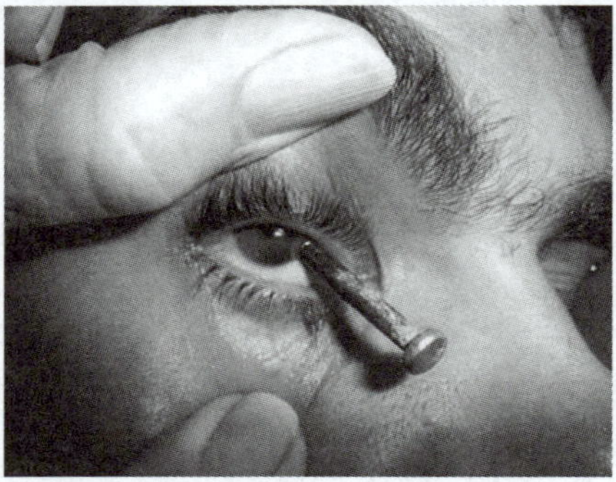

a. Visual acuity test
b. Removal of foreign body
c. Primary survey
d. Antibiotics

Ans. b. Removal of foreign body

Initial Evaluation of Ophthalmic Trauma

Initial evaluation starts with an assessment of the patient's overall condition to identify and manage any life-threatening problems. Then the circumstances of the injury must be established. The patient's level of consciousness may be altered due to substance abuse, psychiatric disease or brain injury, so family members or bystanders may provide crucial collateral information. Specific questions should include whether a blunt or sharp object inflicted the injury; whether the injury occurred at high or low velocity; whether the patient has any prior history of ocular disease or surgery; and when and what the patient last ate and drank.

The next step is ophthalmic examination, of which the extent will depend on the patient's level of cooperation. The first part does not require significant cooperation and begins with an inspection of the eyes and periorbital tissues for any obvious abnormalities such as lacerations, ecchymosis, proptosis, corneal clouding, or gross hyphema. In severe ophthalmic trauma, it is critical to examine the eye as atraumatically as possible to avoid exacerbating the damage. The pupils are examined to determine their absolute and relative sizes and shapes and their responses to direct and consensual illumination. If the patient is conscious and cooperative, visual acuity and confrontation visual fields are tested. Keep in mind that the patient may have broken or lost his or her glasses during the trauma. A pinhole for distance acuity and/or near vision chart and presbyopic reading glasses may be crucial.

If the initial evaluation reveals an injury that warrants further evaluation, ophthalmology consultation is essential. In the presence of a foreign body penetrating into the globe, no attempt should be made to remove the material prior to ophthalmic consultation, as it may lead to leakage of intraocular contents. In addition to reviewing the history, the ophthalmologist will perform an external examination, reassess visual acuity and pupillary responses to light, assess ocular position in each orbit, evaluate ocular alignment and motility, if possible perform slit lamp examination of the anterior segment and measure intraocular pressure, and perform indirect ophthalmoscopy of the fundus.

Further management includes topical antibiotic while there is a corneal epithelial defect; topical cycloplegic to reduce discomfort; topical steroid to reduce inflammation.

3. Which of the following investigations needs to be done for the initial evaluation of a child presenting with the following ocular symptom?

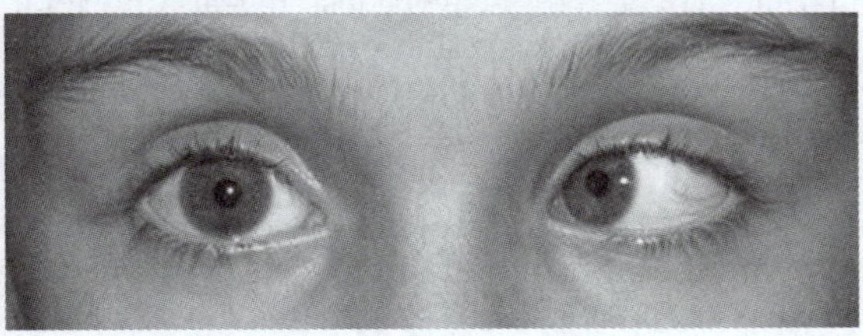

a. Forced duction test
b. Cover uncover test
c. Fundus examination
d. Slit lamp examination

Ans. b. Cover uncover test

Determination of Angle of Deviation in Strabismus

Cover Testing

All four components of cover testing, (1) the cover test, (2) the uncover test, (3) the alternate cover test, and (4) the prism and alternate cover test, require fixation of a target, which may be in any direction of gaze at distance or near.

The cover test identifies manifest strabismus. As the examiner observes one eye, a cover is placed in front of the fellow eye to block its view of the target. If the observed eye moves to take up fixation, it was not previously fixing the target, and a manifest strabismus is present. The direction of movement is in the opposite direction to the deviation. Childhood strabismus is usually comitant, meaning that the magnitude of the manifest strabismus is not significantly influenced by which eye is fixing or the direction of gaze.

The uncover test provides information on fixation preference if there is manifest strabismus, or identifies latent strabismus if there is no manifest strabismus. As the cover is removed from the eye following the cover test, the eye emerging from under the cover is observed by the examiner. If the position of the eye changes, then either (1) a manifest strabismus is present and the eye is once again taking up fixation indicating that it is the preferred eye, or (2) interruption of binocular vision has allowed the eye to deviate and a latent strabismus is revealed. In either case, the direction of corrective movement indicates the type of manifest or latent strabismus, with the same pattern as in the cover test (e.g., outward movement reveals esotropia or esophoria). In manifest strabismus, there will also be a movement of the fellow eye. In latent strabismus, there will be no movement of the fellow eye. If the uncover test results in no movement of the uncovered eye, then either (1) a manifest strabismus is present but the fellow eye has maintained fixation, indicating alternating fixation, or (2) orthophoria (absence of any manifest or latent strabismus) is present, but this is rarely seen clinically.

The alternate cover (cross-cover) test reveals the total deviation (manifest plus latent strabismus). The cover is placed alternately in front of one eye and then the other. It should be moved rapidly from one eye to the other to prevent re-fusion of a latent strabismus.

The prism and alternate cover test quantifies strabismus. Increasing strength of prism is placed in front of one eye oriented with apex toward the deviation until there is neutralization of the movement on alternate cover testing.

4. The following test is used for the assessment of:

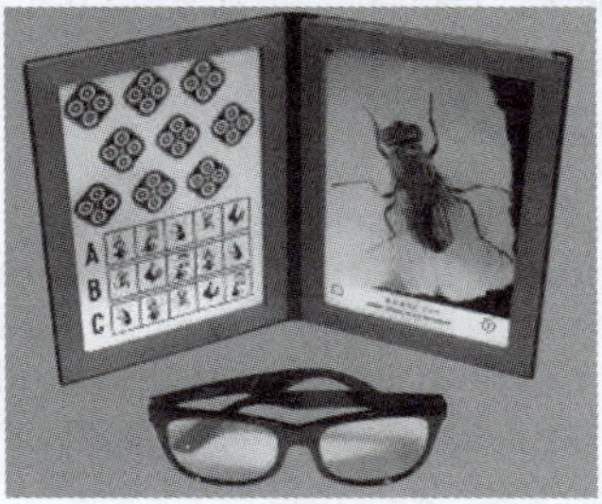

a. Stereopsis
b. Color vision
c. Visual field
d. Visual acuity

Ans. a. Stereopsis

Binocular Vision and Stereopsis Testing

Binocular vision can be subdivided into simultaneous perception, fusion (which requires sensory and motor fusion), and stereopsis. Tests for simultaneous perception and fusion involve presentation of a different stimulus to each eye, such as with red/green or polarized glasses, and analysis of how well the stimuli can be fused. Stereopsis is measured by the same technique using animal figures (e.g., Titmus/Wirt Fly), shapes (e.g., Frisby), or random dot stereograms (TNO, Randot), with the necessary disparity between the images for a three-dimensional form to be seen if stereopsis is present. The images can be presented with a haploscopic system (synoptophore), which, along with random dot stereograms, most effectively minimizes monocular depth clues.

5. What is the abnormality depicted in the following image?

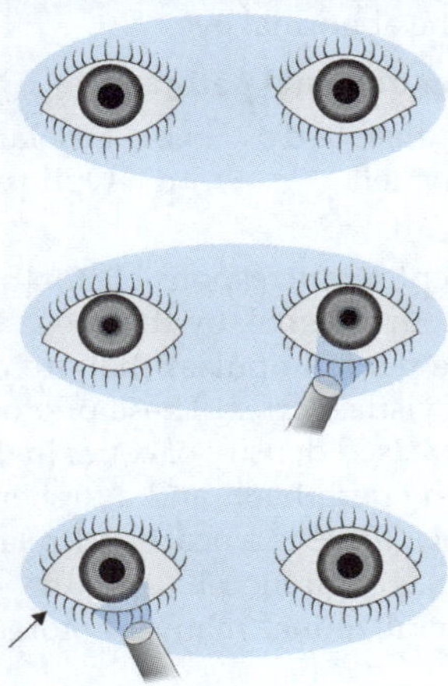

a. Marcus Gunn pupil
b. Optic neuritis
c. Argyll Robertson pupil
d. Pin point pupil

Ans. a. Marcus Gunn pupil

Afferent Pupillary Defect

One of the most important assessments in a patient complaining of decreased vision is whether it is due to an ocular problem (e.g., cataract) or to a potentially more serious optic nerve problem. If an optic nerve lesion is present, the pupillary light response (both the direct response in the stimulated eye and the consensual response in the fellow eye) is less intense when the involved eye is stimulated than when the normal eye is stimulated. This phenomenon is called a relative afferent pupillary defect (RAPD)/ Marcus Gunn pupil. It is made more obvious by alternate stimulation of one eye then the other ensuring that the intensity and duration of stimulation of each eye are the same (swinging penlight test). It will be present also if there is a large retinal or severe macular lesion, but even dense cataract does not impair the pupillary light response. Other causes of unilateral decreased vision without an RAPD include refractive error, media opacity other than cataract such as corneal opacity or vitreous hemorrhage, amblyopia, and functional visual loss. In a lesion of the brachium of the superior colliculus, it is possible for an RAPD to be present when visual function is normal.

Absolute afferent pupillary defect is the absence of pupillary response to light stimulation of a completely blind (amaurotic) eye. Light shone into the normal eye would still induce a consensual response in the blind eye.

An afferent pupillary defect can still be identified if one pupil is either not visible, due to corneal disease, or is unable to respond due to structural damage or damage to its innervation, for example, third nerve palsy, by examination of the normal pupil as light is shone into the normal and then into the abnormal eye.

6. First order neuron of visual pathway is:

a. Lateral geniculate body
b. Bipolar neuron
c. Photoreceptor cell
d. Optic nerve

Ans. c. Photoreceptor cell

Rod and cone photoreceptors are responsible for the initial transformation of light stimulus into neural signal, by the process of phototransduction of light stimuli into the nerve impulses that are conducted through the visual pathways to the visual cortex. These photoreceptors are arranged such that there is an increased density of cones in the center of the macula (fovea), decreasing to the periphery, and a higher density of rods in the periphery. In the foveola, there is a nearly 1:1 relationship between each cone photoreceptor, its ganglion cell, and the emerging nerve fiber, whereas in the peripheral retina, many photoreceptors connect to the same ganglion cell.

Transmission of neural signals in various layers of retina:

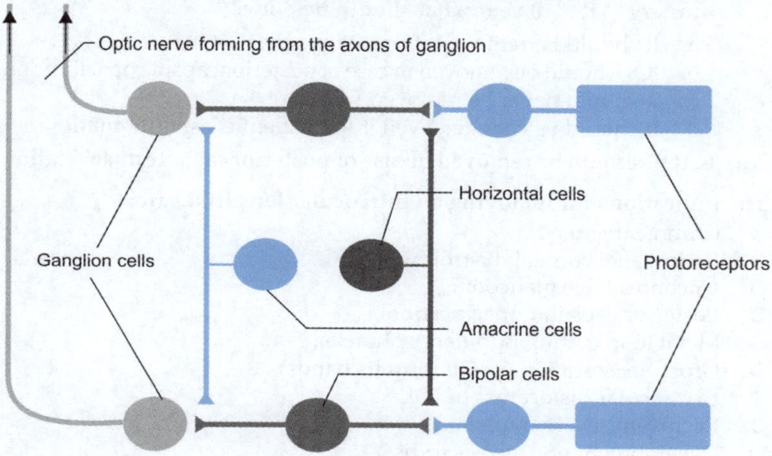

The optic pathway:

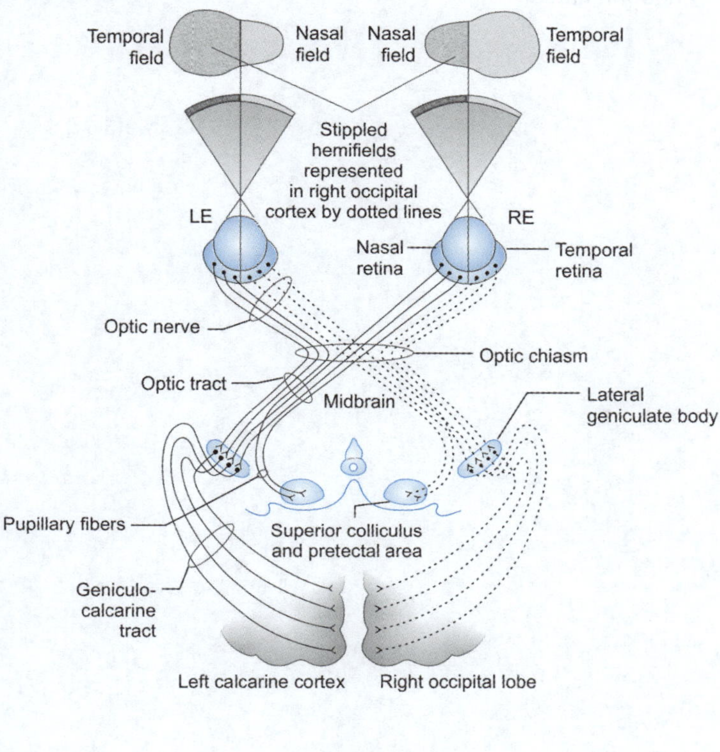

7. An IOL has been placed in a young male following cataract surgery. After 10 year what should be done?

a. It should be removed if presbyopia has set in
b. IOL should be removed in case of posterior capsule opacification
c. It should never be removed
d. It should be changed even if the patient is asymptomatic

Ans. **b. IOL should be removed in case of posterior capsule opacification**

The indications for removing an intraocular lens (IOL) are:

- Chronic uveitis
- Endothelial corneal dystrophy
- Uncontrollable glaucoma
- Posterior capsular opacification
- Metal loop cutting pupillary sphincter
- Gross decentration of IOL (fibrous bands)
- Extraocular dislocation of IOL.
- Recurrent severe hyphema
- Development of rubeosis iridis
- Removal of iris in case of - (1) Iris tumor (2) Epithelial downgrowth
- Endophthalmitis

ENT

1. A patient presented to the ENT OPD with left sided hearing loss. Audiogram revealed the following findings. What is the most likely diagnosis?

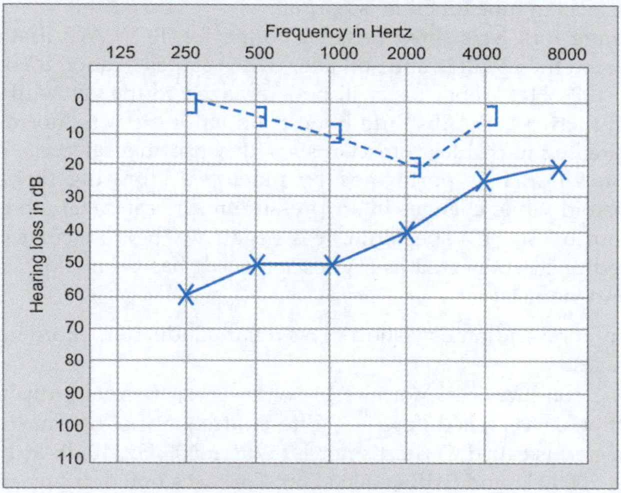

a. Otosclerosis
b. Schwannoma
c. Perilymph fistula
d. Meniere's disease

Ans. 'a' Otosclerosis

Otosclerosis

It is a primary disease of the bony labyrinth. In this, one or more foci of irregularly laid spongy bone replace part of normally dense endochondral layer of bony otic capsule.

Symptoms

- *Hearing loss*: This is the presenting symptom and usually starts in twenties. It is painless and progressive with insidious onset. Often it is bilateral conductive type.
- *Paracusis Willisii*: An otosclerotic patient hears better in noisy than in quiet surroundings. This is because a normal person will raise his voice in noisy surroundings.
- *Tinnitus*: It is more commonly seen in cochlear otosclerosis and in active lesions.
- *Vertigo*: It is an uncommon symptom.
- *Speech*: Patient has a monotonous, well-modulated soft speech.

Signs

- Tympanic membrane is quite normal and mobile. Sometimes, a reddish hue may be seen on the promontory through the tympanic membrane (Schwartze sign). This is indicative of active focus with increased vascularity.
- Eustachian tube function is normal.
- Tuning fork tests show negative Rinne (i.e. BC > AC) first for 256 Hz and then 512 Hz and still later, when stapes fixation is complete, for 1026 Hz. Weber test will be lateralized to the ear with greater conductive loss. Absolute bone conduction may be normal. It is decreased in cochlear otosclerosis with sensorineural loss.
- *Gelle's test*: It is performed by placing a vibrating fork on the mastoid while changes in air pressure in the car canal are brought about by Siegle's speculum. It is negative when ossicular chain is fixed or disconnected as in otosclerosis. It has been superseded by tympanometry.

Pure tone audiometry shows loss of air conduction, more for lower frequencies.

Bone conduction is normal. In some cases, there is a dip in bone conduction curve. It is different at different frequencies but maximum at 2000 Hz and is called Carhart's notch (5 dB at 500 Hz, 10 dB at 1000 Hz, 15 dB at 2000 Hz and 5 dB at 4000 Hz). Carhart's notch disappears after successful stapedectomy.

Cahart's Notch

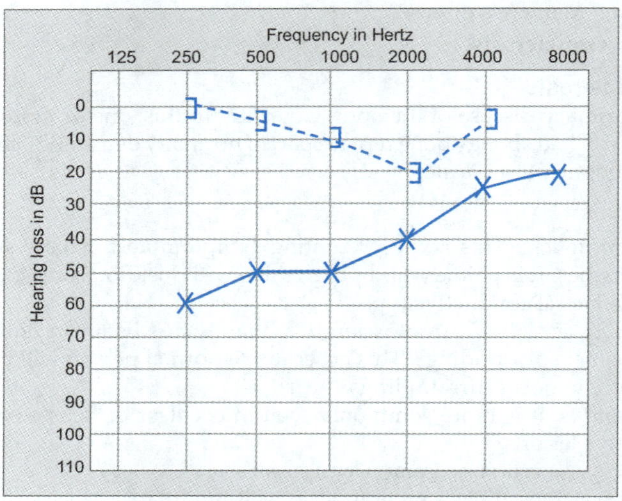

Mixed hearing loss is not uncommon in otosclerosis.

Speech audiometry reveals normal discrimination score except in those with cochlear involvement.

Tympanometry may be normal in early cases but later shows a curve of ossicular stiffness. Stapedial reflex becomes absent when stapes is fixed.

Treatment of Otosclerosis

- *Medical*: There is no medical treatment that cures otosclerosis. Sodium fluoride has been tried to hasten the maturity of active focus and arrest further cochlear loss, but controversies exist and this treatment is not recommended generally.
- *Surgical*: Stapedectomy/stapedotomy with a placement of prosthesis is the treatment of choice. Here the fixed otosclerotic stapes is removed and a prosthesis inserted between the incus and oval window. Prosthesis employed may be a teflon piston, stainless steel piston, platinum–Teflon or titanium–teflon piston. In 90% of patients, there is good improvement in hearing after stapedectomy.
- *Selection of patients for stapes surgery*: Hearing threshold for air conduction should be 30 dB or worse. (It is this level when patient starts feeling socially handicapped.) Average air-bone gap should be at least 15 dB with Rinne negative for 256 and 512 Hz. Speech discrimination score should be 60% or more.

2. Arrange the following components of auditory pathway in correct sequence from periphery to centre:

a. Lateral lemniscus
b. Cochlear nerve
c. Medial geniculate body
d. Inferior colliculus

Ans. **b: Cochlear nerve, a: Lateral lemniscus, d: Inferior colliculus, c: Medial geniculate body**

Auditory Pathway

Hair cells are innervated by dendrites of bipolar cells of spiral ganglion which is situated in Rosenthal's canal (canal running along the osseous spiral lamina). Axons of these bipolar cells form the cochlear division of CN VIII and end in the cochlear nuclei, the dorsal and ventral, on each side of the medulla. From cochlear nuclei, the main nuclei in the ascending auditory pathway are:

- Superior olivary complex
- Nucleus of lateral lemniscus
- Inferior colliculus
- Medial geniculate body
- Auditory cortex

The auditory fibres travel via the ipsilateral and contralateral routes and have multiple decussation points. Thus each ear is represented in both cerebral hemispheres. The area of cortex, concerned with hearing is situated in the superior temporal gyrus (Brodmann's area 41).

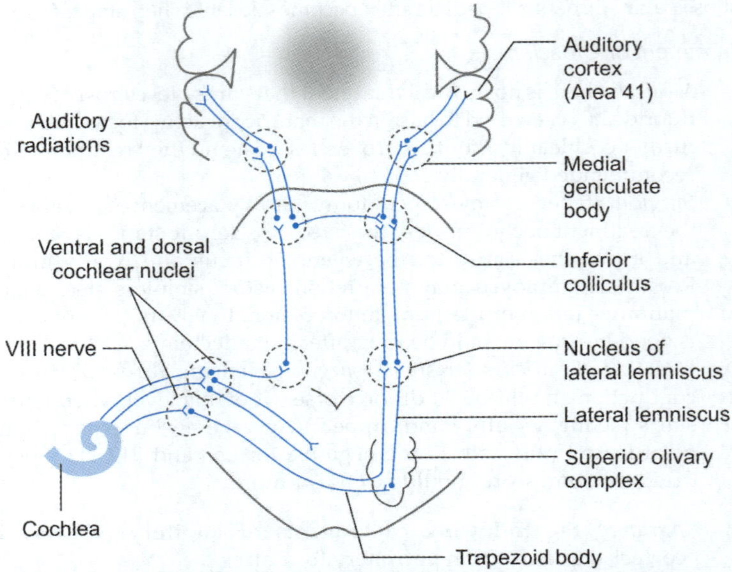

3. All are risk factors for head and neck SCC, *except*:

a. HIV
b. Vitamin A deficiency
c. Betel nut
d. EBV

Ans. a. HIV

Risk Factors for Head and Neck Cancers

- *Smoking*: It is the single most important risk factor. In certain parts of India, there is an unusual habit of reverse smoking where burning end of the "churat" (rolled tobacco leaf) is put in the mouth. This gives high incidence of cancer of the hard palate.
- *Tobacco chewing*: Powdered tobacco, mixed with lime, is placed in some part of the vestibule of the mouth. Carcinoma develops at the site of the quid. Chewing "pan" and keeping the quid in the vestibule is largely responsible for oral cancer in India.
- *Alcohol*: Cancer of upper aerodigestive tract occurs six times more in heavy drinkers as compared to nondrinkers.

- *Dietary deficiencies*: Vitamin A and Riboflavin deficiency are implicated as risk factors for oral cavity cancers.
- *Prolonged sun exposure*: This is especially linked to cancer in the lip area, as well as skin cancer of the head and neck.
- *Human papillomavirus (HPV)*: Sexual activity with a person who has HPV is the most common way someone gets HPV. Certain strains of HPV have been implicated as risk factor for oral cavity cancers.
- *Epstein-Barr virus (EBV)*: Exposure to EBV, plays a role in the development of nasopharyngeal cancer.
- *Gender*: Men are 2 to 3 times more likely than women to develop head and neck cancer.
- *Age*: People over the age of 40 are at higher risk for head and neck cancer.
- *Environmental or occupational inhalants*: Inhaling asbestos, wood dust, paint fumes, and certain chemicals may increase a person's risk of head and neck cancer.
- *Gastroesophageal reflux disease (GERD) and laryngopharyngeal reflux disease (LPRD)*: Reflux of stomach acid into the upper airway and throat has been suggested as a factor associated with the development of head and neck cancer.
- Paterson–Brown–Kelly syndrome also called Plummer–Vinson syndrome (iron deficiency anaemia) is responsible for cancer of the oral cavity and hypopharynx.
- Dental sepsis, jagged sharp teeth and ill-fitting dentures.

4. Which of the following arteries supplying the nasal septum is not a branch of ECA?

a. Anterior ethmoidal artery
b. Sphenopalatine artery
c. Greater palatine artery
d. Superior labial artery

Ans. **a. Anterior ethmoidal artery**

Blood Supply of Nasal Septum

Little's area and Kiesselbach's plexus:

It is situated in the anterior inferior part of nasal septum, just above the vestibule. Four arteries—anterior ethmoidal, septal branch of superior labial, septal branch of sphenopalatine and the greater palatine, anastomose here to form a vascular plexus called "Kiesselbach's plexus." This area is exposed to the drying effect of inspiratory current and to finger nail trauma, and is the usual site for epistaxis in children and young adults.

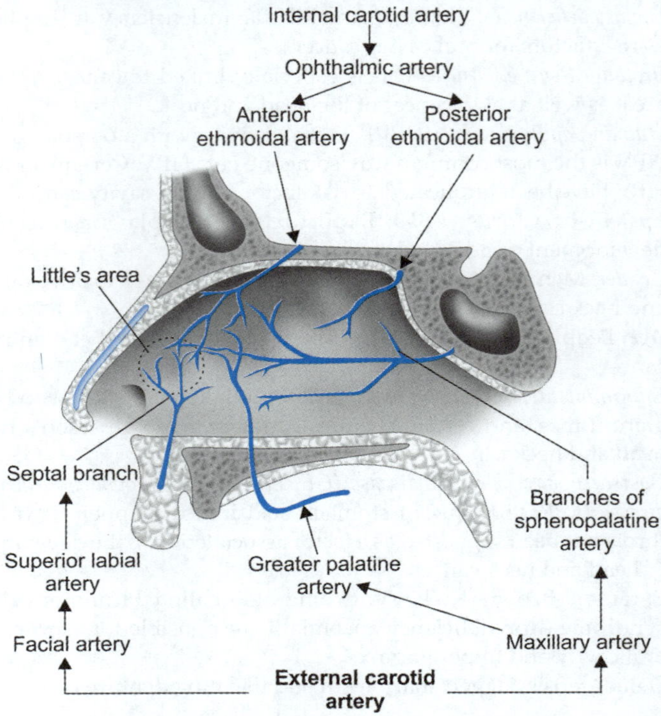
Internal carotid artery
Ophthalmic artery
Anterior ethmoidal artery
Posterior ethmoidal artery
Little's area
Septal branch
Superior labial artery
Facial artery
Greater palatine artery
Branches of sphenopalatine artery
Maxillary artery
External carotid artery

Preventive and Social Medicine

1. Mw vaccine is made from which bacteria?

a. *M. welchii*
b. *M. indicus pranii*
c. *M. avium intracellulare*
d. None of the above

Ans. b. *M. indicus pranii*

- Killed Mycobacterium *indicus pranii* (previously known as Mycobacterium w, popularly known as Mw) vaccine has been approved by the Drug Controller General of India. It is being rolled out in a project involving five districts in the states of Bihar and Gujarat, where there are high rates of leprosy.
- People affected by leprosy as well as their families and other people who come into close contact with them on a regular basis, such as colleagues, will benefit from the project, making India the first country in the world to have a large-scale leprosy vaccination initiative.
- They will be given the vaccine, *mycobacterium indicus pranii* (MIP), in combination with a single dose of the drug rifampicin, which is already being trialled in several countries to prevent leprosy in those who have been exposed to family members who already have the disease. A recent study by The Leprosy Mission in Bangladesh found that new leprosy cases among people who had been given a single dose of rifampicin were almost 60% fewer than among those who had been given a placebo.
- Mycobacterium w vaccine, is also useful adjuvant to multidrug therapy in multibacillary leprosy.

2. Transmission assessment survey is for:

a. *P. vivax*
b. *P. falciparum*
c. *Leishmania donovani*
d. *Wuchereria Bancrofti*

Ans. d. *Wuchereria Bancrofti*

Lymphatic Filariasis Transmission Assessment Survey

The Transmission Assessment Survey (TAS) for lymphatic filariasis is conducted to determine whether infection has been reduced to levels below which transmission is no longer sustainable, allowing for a decision to stop mass drug administration (MDA). The same strategy is also used for surveillance after stopping MDA to ensure that recrudescence is not occurring.

3. All of the following statements are true about AFP surveillance *except*:

a. It should be carried out for adults if there is suspicion of polio
b. It should not be carried out for children < 5 years of age
c. AFP greater than 1/100,000 population is good functional surveillance
d. Once diagnosed follow-up should be carried out till 60 days after the detection

Ans. **b. It should not be carried out for children < 5 years of age**

Acute Flaccid Paralysis Surveillance

There are four steps of acute flaccid paralysis (AFP) surveillance:

1. *Finding and reporting children with acute flaccid paralysis (AFP)*: Healthcare staff must promptly report every case of acute flaccid paralysis {AFP) in any child under 15 years of age. Any child under 15 years of age with AFP or any person of any age with paralytic illness if polio is suspected is included. In addition, public health staff make regular visits to hospitals and rehabilitation centres to search for AFP cases which may have been overlooked or misdiagnosed. The number of AFP cases reported each year is used as an indicator of a country's ability to detect polio even in countries where the disease no longer occurs. A country's surveillance system needs to be sensitive enough to detect at least one case of AFP for every 100,000 children under 15 years even in the absence of polio. At least 80% of AFP cases should have a follow-up examination for residual paralysis at 60 days after the onset of paralysis.
2. *Transporting stool samples for analysis*: In the early stages, polio may be difficult to differentiate from other forms of acute flaccid paralysis, such as Guillain-Barre Syndrome, transverse myelitis, or traumatic neuritis. All children with acute flaccid paralysis (AFP) should be reported and tested for wild poliovirus within 48 hours of onset, even if doctors are confident on clinical grounds that the child does not have polio. To test for polio, fecal specimens are analyzed for the presence of poliovirus. Because shedding of the virus is variable, two specimens taken 24–48 hours apart are required. Speed is essential, since the highest concentrations of poliovirus in the stools of infected individuals are found during the first two weeks after onset of paralysis. Stool specimens have to be sealed in containers and stored immediately inside a refrigerator or packed between frozen ice packs at 4–8°C in a cold box, ready for shipment to a laboratory. Undue delays or prolonged exposure to heat on the way to the laboratory may destroy the virus. Specimens should arrive at the laboratory within 72 hours of collection.
3. *Isolating poliovirus*: In a laboratory, virologists begin the task of isolating poliovirus from the stool samples. If poliovirus is isolated,

the next step is to distinguish between wild (naturally occurring) and vaccine-related poliovirus. This is necessary because the oral vaccine consists of attenuated live polioviruses and resembles wild virus in the laboratory. If wild poliovirus is isolated, the virologists identify which of the two surviving types of wild virus is involved. Wild poliovirus type 2 has not been recorded since 1999.

4. *Mapping the virus*: Once wild poliovirus has been identified, further tests are carried out to determine where the strain may have originated. By determining the exact genetic make-up of the virus, wild viruses can be compared to others and classified into genetic families which cluster in defined geographical areas. The newly-found poliovirus sequence is checked against a reference bank of known polioviruses, allowing inferences about the geographical origin of the newly found virus. When polio has been pinpointed to a precise geographical area, it is possible to identify the source of importation of poliovirus – both long-range and cross-border. Appropriate immunization strategies can then be determined to prevent further spread of the poliovirus.

4. All of the following done to remove confounders *except*:

a. Randomization
b. Restriction
c. Random selection
d. Matching

Ans. c. Random selection

Confounding occurs when there is a third variable that is independently linked to both the risk factor and the disease outcome under study. For example, epidemiologic studies published a number of years ago reported an association between consumption of coffee and the development of certain types of cancer. However, it was subsequently shown that the findings were confounded by failure to control for cigarette smoking. Those individuals who drink coffee are also more likely to smoke, and smoking is an independent risk factor for cancer. Although the investigators thought they were comparing groups who differed in the amount of coffee consumed, in reality, they were comparing groups with differing numbers of cigarettes consumed, and it was this latter risk factor that resulted in the observed difference in cancer between the groups.

Confounding can be handled using a variety of approaches. However, it is obvious that to control a confounder, one must be aware of it. The only method available to control for unknown confounders is randomization in a clinical trial. With appropriate randomization, groups will be the same with respect to every variable, including both known and unknown confounders, and differ only with respect to the intervention under study.

Methods to Control Confounding

Method	Example	Limitation
Matching	For each case with disease, a control is selected with the same level of confounder	Does not allow any measurement of the strength of the confounder
Stratification	Divide subjects into different levels of the confounder	Only practical for a small number of confounders
Randomization	Randomly allocate subjects to receive the intervention under study	Requires control of the intervention on the part of investigators
Multivariate analysis	Control influence of other variables using statistical software to isolate and examine the effect of one	Methods are complex
Restriction	A study of cardiovascular disease only enrolls men	Reduces the generalizability of the study findings

5. Which of the following vaccines is/are effective for mass vaccination during a disaster outbreak?

a. Cholera
b. Typhoid
c. Measles
d. Scrub typhus

Ans. a-F, b-F, c-F, d-F

Vaccination During Outbreak of a Disaster

Health authorities are often under considerable public and political pressure to begin mass vaccination programmes, usually against typhoid, cholera and tetanus. The WHO does not recommend typhoid and cholera vaccines in routine use in endemic areas. The newer typhoid and cholera vaccines have increased efficacy, but because they are multidose vaccines, compliance is likely to be poor. They have not yet been proven effective, as a large-scale public health measure. Vaccination programme requires large number of workers who could be better employed elsewhere. Supervision of sterilization and injection techniques may be impossible, resulting in more harm than good. And above all, mass vaccination may lead to false sense of security about the risk of the disease and to the neglect of effective control measures. However, these vaccinations are recommended for health workers.

Supplying safe drinking water and proper disposal of excreta continue to be the most practical and effective strategy. Significant increase in tetanus incidence have not occurred after natural disasters. Mass vaccination of population against tetanus is usually unnecessary. The best protection is maintenance of a high level of immunity in the general population by routine vaccination before the disaster occurs, and adequate wound cleaning and treatment.

6. In a village with a population of 20000, 456 babies were born in a year, out of which 56 died before 28 weeks. 34 more died within 1 year. Total no of deaths in the village were 500. Calculate the IMR:

a. 4.5
b. 123
c. 197
d. 18

Ans. c. 197

Infant mortality rate = (Number of infant deaths (< 1 year of age)/ Number of live births) x 1000

Number of infant deaths = 56 + 34 = 90

Number of live births = 456

Therefore, IMR = (90/456) × 1000

= 0.197 × 100

= 197

7. Which of the following national health programmes aims at improving the quality of care in labour rooms?

a. LaQshya
b. JSSK
c. Ayushman Bharat
d. Janani Suraksha Yojna

Ans. a. LaQshya

LaQshya' programme of the Ministry of Health and Family Welfare aims at improving quality of care in labour room and maternity operation theatre (OT).

Goal

Reduce preventable maternal and newborn mortality, morbidity and stillbirths associated with the care around delivery in labour room and Maternity OT and ensure respectful maternity care.

Objectives

To reduce maternal and newborn mortality and morbidity due to APH, PPH, retained placenta, preterm, preeclampsia and eclampsia, obstructed labour, puerperal sepsis, newborn asphyxia, and sepsis, etc.

To improve Quality of care during the delivery and immediate post-partum care, stabilization of complications and ensure timely referrals, and enable an effective two-way follow-up system.

To enhance satisfaction of beneficiaries visiting the health facilities and provide Respectful Maternity Care (RMC) to all pregnant women attending the public health facility.

Strategies

Reorganizing/aligning Labour room and Maternity Operation Theatre layout and workflow as per 'Labour Room Standardization Guidelines' and 'Maternal and Newborn Health Toolkit' issued by the Ministry of Health & Family Welfare, Government of India.

Ensuring that at least all government medical college hospitals and high case-load district hospitals have dedicated obstetric HDUs as per GoI MOHFW Guidelines, for managing complicated pregnancies that require life-saving critical care.

Ensuring strict adherence to clinical protocols for management and stabilization of the complications before referral to higher centres.

8. During a survey at a subcentre, the mean diastolic blood pressure of the population was 110 mm Hg with standard deviation of 11 while the mean vitamin D level was 18 ng/mL with standard deviation of 3. Which one of the following statements is true?

a. Diastolic blood pressure is more variable
b. Vitamin D level is more variable
c. Both are equally variable
d. Data inconclusive

Ans. **b. Vitamin D level is more variable**

Coefficient of Variation

The coefficient of variation (CV) is a measure of relative variability. It is the ratio of the standard deviation to the mean (average). The CV is particularly useful while comparing results from two different surveys or tests that have different measures or values.

The formula for the coefficient of variation is:

Coefficient of Variation = (Standard deviation/Mean) x 100.

In the given question, because we need to compare variables with different unit and mean, CV needs to be calculated. On calculation, CV of BP would be 10%, while that of vitamin D level would be 16.7%. Therefore, vitamin D level is more variable than diastolic BP.

9. A study was conducted to test the efficacy of a new vaccine in preventing a particular disease in a population. The incidence of the disease before and after the introduction of vaccine were compared for the same. Which of the following tests would you use for statistical analysis?

a. Chi-square test
b. Unpaired t test
c. Paired t test
d. Regression analysis

Ans. **c. Paired t test**

In the given question, we have to assess the incidence of the disease before and after administration of the vaccine, which is repeat measurement in the same group. Hence, paired t test is the most appropriate test.

Tests of Significance

Number of groups	Parametric areas	Nonparametric areas
Independent measures, 2 groups	Unpaired t-test or Student t-test	Chi-square test (large or small sample with Yate's correction) Fischer's test (small or large sample) Mann-Whitney U-test (Wilcoxon Rank sum test)
Independent measures, > 2 groups	ANOVA	Kruskal-Wallis test Chi-square test
Repeated measures, 2 conditions or paired data	Paired t-test	Wilcoxon signed rank test, Mc-Nemar's test Chi-square test
Repeated measures, > 2 conditions	ANOVA	Friedman's test Chi-square test
Correlation test	Pearson	Spearman (Rho)
Regression	Simple linear or nonlinear regression	Nonparametric regression

10. Match the following:

Column 1	Column 2
A. Yellow bag	1. Gloves
B. Red bag	2. Glassware
C. Blue bag	3. Syringe wrapper
D. White transparent container	4. Scalpel
	5. Chemical waste

Ans. A-5, B-1, C-2, D-4

Biomedical Waste Management

Cat.	Type of Bag/ Container used	Type of waste	Treatment/ disposal options
Yellow	➢ Non-chlorinated plastic bags ➢ Separate collection system leading to effluent treatment system	➢ Human anatomical waste ➢ Animal anatomical waste ➢ Soiled waste ➢ Expired or discarded medicines ➢ Chemical waste ➢ Microbiological and other clinical lab waste including blood bags ➢ Chemical liquid waste	➢ Incineration or plasma ➢ Pyrolysis or deep burial

Contd...

Contd...

Cat.	Type of Bag/ Container used	Type of waste	Treatment/ disposal options
Red	Non-chlorinated plastic bags or containers	Contaminated waste (Recyclable) tubing, bottles, intravenous tubes and sets, catheters, urine bags, syringes (without needles) and gloves.	Auto/micro/ hydro and then sent for recycling. Not be sent to landfill
White	(Translucent) Puncture, leak, tamper proof containers	Waste sharps including metals	Auto or dry heat sterilizations followed by shredding or mutilation or encapsulation
Blue	Cardboard boxes with blue colored marking	Glassware	Disinfection or auto/micro/ hydro and then sent for recycling

11. Mark the following statements are true or false with regards to responsibilities of ASHA worker:

a. Prepare blood slide for malaria
b. Perform immunization as per schedule
c. Taking pregnant mother to hospital
d. Counsel the mother on safe breastfeeding practices

Ans. a-F, b-F, c-T, d-T

Accredited Social Health Activist (ASHA)

Selection of ASHA: ASHA must be the resident of the village—a woman (married/widow/divorced) preferably in the age group of 25 to 45 years with formal education up to eighth class, having communication skills and leadership qualities. Adequate representation from the disadvantaged population group will ensure to serve such groups better.

The general norm of selection is one ASHA for 1000 population. In tribal, hilly and desert areas the norm could be relaxed to one ASHA per habitation.

Roles and Responsibilities

1. ASHA will take steps to create awareness and provide information to the community on determinants of health such as nutrition, basic sanitation and hygienic practices, healthy living and working conditions, information on existing health services, and the need for timely utilization of health and family welfare services.
2. She will counsel women on birth preparedness, importance of safe delivery, breastfeeding and complementary feeding, immunization. contraception and prevention of common infections including

reproductive tract infection/sexually transmitted infection and care of the young child.

3. ASHA will mobilize the community and facilitate them in accessing health and health-related services available at the anganwadi/ subcentre/primary health centres, such as immunization, antenatal check-up, postnatal check-up, supplementary nutrition, sanitation and other services being provided by the government.
4. She will work with the village health and sanitation committee of the gram panchayat to develop a comprehensive village health plan.
5. She will arrange escort/accompany pregnant women and children requiring treatment/admission to the nearest pre-identified health facility i.e. primary health centre/community health centre/First Referral Unit.
6. ASHA will provide primary medical care for minor ailments such as diarrhea, fevers, and first-aid for minor injuries. She will be a provider of directly observed treatment short-course (DOTS).
7. She will also act as a depot holder for essential provisions being made available to every habitation like oral rehydration therapy, iron folic acid tablet, chloroquine, disposable delivery kits, oral pills and condoms etc.
8. She will inform about the births and deaths in her village and any unusual health problems/disease outbreaks in the community to the sub-centre/primary health centre.

12. Which of the following diseases is NOT transmitted by it?

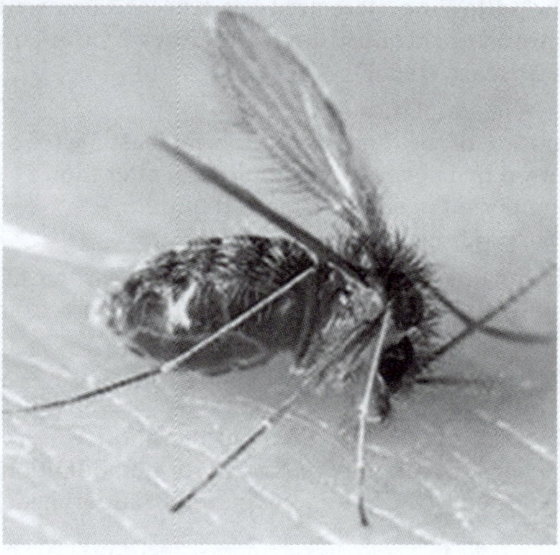

a. Kala Azar b. Chandipur encephalitis
c. Carrion's disease
d. Babesiosis

Ans. d. Babesiosis

The given image is that of a sandfly

Sand-fly

Sandflies act as vector for the following diseases

- Phlebotamusargentipes - Kala-Azar
- Phlebolamuspapatasii - Sandfly fever
- Phlebotamussergenti - Oriental sore
- Chandipur encephalitis
- Carrion disease/Oroya fever

Morphology

Adults are about 1.5–3.0 mm long and yellowish in color, with conspicuous black eyes, hairy bodies, wings and legs.

- The oval lanceolate wings are carried erect on the humped thorax.
- Males possess long prominent genital terminalia known as claspers. Females have a pair of anal recti.
- Only female sandfly can bite in the dwelling at night.
- It takes shelter during day in holes and crevices in wall, in dark room and store room, etc.

Dispersal: Range of flight is 200 yard from their breeding places.

Life span: Average life of sandfly is about 2 weeks.

13. Mark the following statements as true or false with regards to the definition of chronic illness laid down by the Commission on Chronic Disease (1956)?

a. Leave residual disability
b. Duration of the illness should be at least 3 weeks
c. Caused by irreversible pathological alteration
d. Long period of supervision is required

Ans. a-T, b-F, c-T, d-T

This is a fact based question. The Commission on Chronic Diseases (1956) defines chronic disease as all impairments or deviations from normal that have one or more of the following characteristics:

- Are permanent
- Leave residual disability
- Caused by non-reversible pathologic alteration
- Require special training of the patient for rehabilitation
- May be expected to require a long period of supervision, observation or care

14. A study was conducted to assess the effect of an intervention for certain disease. The p values for two similar researches and B with 95% confidence limits, was found to be 0.02 and 0.001 respectively using text "X" and "Y" with a control group. Based on preliminary analysis, the result may be interpreted as:

A. Study B is more precise than study A and intervention Y is more significant compared to Intervention X for us in community.
B. Study A is more precise than study B and intervention X is more significant compared to Intervention Y for us in community.
C. Both X and Y show a significant variation, but Study B is more significant than study A.
D. Both study A and B shows a significant variation and both interventions have similar statistically significance.
E. Data is not sufficient to compare the investigations.

a. If A, B, C are correct
b. If A and C are correct
c. If B and D are correct
d. If all four (A, B, C, & D) are correct

Ans. **b. If A and C are correct**

- **Interpretation of p-value**
- P-value helps to determine the significance of results of any study.
- The P-value, or calculated probability, is the probability of finding the observed, or more extreme, results when the null hypothesis (H0) of a study question is true
- Null hypothesis is rejected in favor of alternative if p-value is less than Alpha error (predetermined level of significance)
- P-value in no way tells about the probability of blood pressure reduction, it is just the measure of confidence with which we can state our result.
- The p-value is a number between O and 1 and interpreted in the following way:
- A small p-value (typically <0.05) indicates strong evidence against the null hypothesis, so you reject the null hypothesis.
- A large p-value (>0.05) indicates weak evidence against the null hypothesis, so you fail to reject the null hypothesis.
- p-value very close to the cutoff (0.05) are considered to be marginal.
- Apply the logic; among 0.2 and 0.001 the 0.001 is lies farther and away from the normal disturbance curve. So 0.001 is highly significant p-valve or precise valve and 0.2 is significant p-valve or precise valve. Hence Study B is more precise than study A and intervention Y is more significant compared to Intervention X for us in community.

15. The bone marrow density along with gestational age is plotted from two different researches. Which of the following is true for the relation between bone marrow density and gestational age?

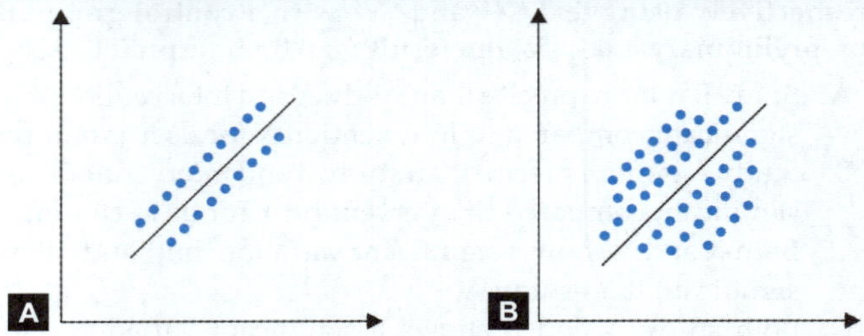

a. Strength of relation is same in A and B
b. Strength of the relation is more in A than in B
c. Strength of the variation is more in B than A
d. Variation in variables is more with A than B

Ans. b. Strength of the relation is more in A than in B

Correlation

- Positive correlation
  - If x & y have a strong positive linear correlation, r is close to + 1.
  - An r value of exactly +1 indicates a perfect positive fit.
  - Positive values indicate a relationship between x and y variables such that as values for x increases, values for y also increase.
- No correlation:
  - If there is no linear correlation or a weak linear correlation, r is close to 0.
  - A value near zero means that there is a random, nonlinear relationship between the two variables.
- Negative correlation:
  - If x & y have a strong negative linear correlation, r is close to −1
  - An r value of exactly −1 indicates a perfect negative fit.
  - Negative values indicate a relationship between x and y such that as values for x increase, values for y decrease.

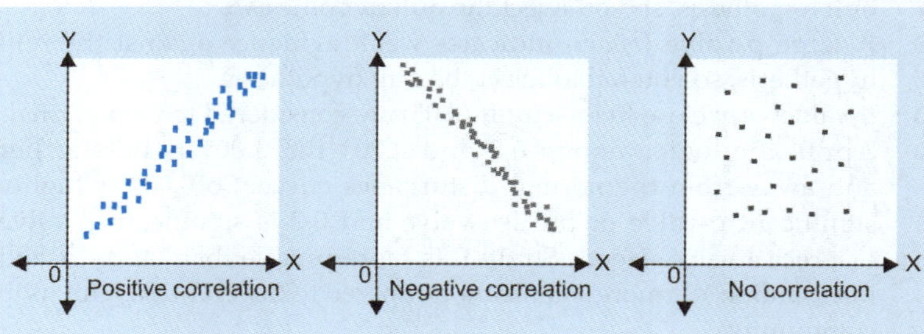

- The direction of scatter helps to determine the presence or absence of association.
- In graph-A: The values are just around the curve.
- In graph-B: The values are given in scattered manner and they are not nicely correlated.
- In the two graphs the coefficient of Variable is nonsignificant.
- The graph A has strong correlation compare to B.
- Variation in variables is less with A than B.

16. Look at the image below the correct corresponding:

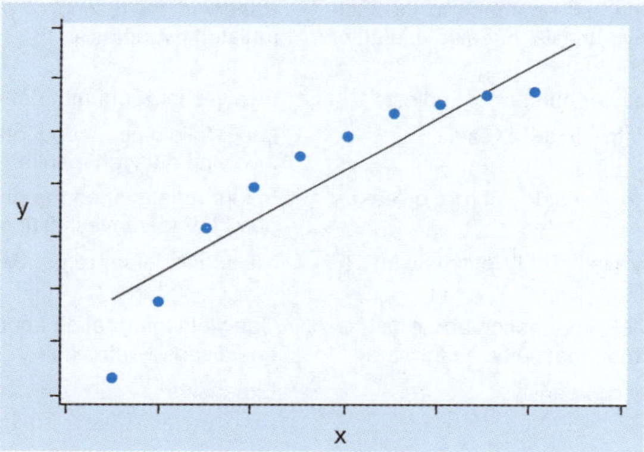

a. y = 10 + x
b. y = 10 + y
c. y = 11 + 2x
d. x = 11 + 2y

Ans. **c. y = 11 + 2x**

- It is a regression analysis graph.
- Regression Equation y = a + bx + e
- y = dependent variable
- a = regression constant or Intercept of slope on y
- b = slope coefficient (slope of the curve)
- x = independent variation
- e = error

17. Which is the study design of choice for finding out circadian variation of fat content in expressed breast milk of mother of preterm babies:

a. Prospective cohort
b. Ambispective cohort
c. Case control
d. Cross sectional

Ans. **a. Prospective cohort**

Types of Observational Studies

Case control study	Cohort study
➤ Proceeds from 'effect to cause'	➤ Proceeds from 'cause to effect'
➤ Starts with the disease	➤ Starts with people exposed to risk factor or suspected cause
➤ Tests whether the suspected cause occurs more frequently in those with the disease than among those without the disease	➤ Tests whether disease occurs more frequently in those exposed, than in those not similarly exposed
➤ Usually the first approach to the testing of a hypothesis, but also useful for exploratory studies	➤ Reserved for testing of precisely formulated hypothesis
➤ Involves fewer number of subjects	➤ Involves larger number of subjects
➤ Yields relatively quick results	➤ Long follow-up period often needed, involving delayed results
➤ Suitable for the study of rare diseases	➤ Inappropriate when the disease or exposure under investigation is rare
➤ Generally yields only estimate of RR (odds ratio)	➤ Yields incidence rates, RR as well as AR
➤ Cannot yield information about diseases other than that selected for study	➤ Can yield information about more than one disease outcome
➤ Relatively inexpensive	➤ Expensive

Cross-sectional Study

- Based on a single examination of a cross-section of population at one point of time
- More useful for chronic rather than short-lived diseases
- Provides information about prevalence (Also known as prevalence study)
- It provides no information about incidence or natural history of disease.

18. A study was conducted to assess the effectiveness of a new treatment for a particular disease. In the control population, there were 36 deaths/treatment failures out of sample of 120. With the new treatment, 26 treatment failure were reported from a sample size of 130. How many patients should be treated to avert a single death?

a. 100
b. 10
c. 250
d. 160

Ans. **b. 10**

The given details can be tabulated as below:

	Treatment failure	No treatment failure	Total
Experimental group	26	104	130
Control group	36	84	120

From the given data, it is clear that incidence of treatment failure with new treatment = 26/130 = 0.2, and

Incidence of adverse outcome without the treatment = 36/120 = 0.3

Absolute risk reduction is the total percentage reduction in incidence of adverse outcome.

So, absolute risk reduction = adverse outcome without the treatment-adverse outcome without the treatment

= 0.3-0.2 = 0.1, which is equal to 10%

This means that if 100 patients are given the treatment, the 10 patients would be benefitted. Extrapolating the same, to avoid adverse outcome for one patient, 10 patients need to be given treatment.

19. A study was done to assess the risk factors for breast cancer in 100 females from urban cities. A statistical group and analysis is shown below. How many risk factors may be ascertained from the statistical analysis of the research?

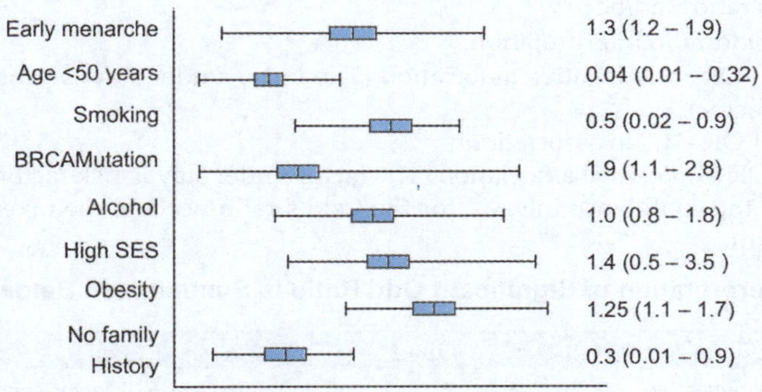

a. 3
b. 4
c. 5
d. 6

Ans. a. 3

Forest Plot

- A forest plot, also known as a blobbogram, is a graphical display of estimated results from a number of scientific studies addressing the same question, along with the overall results.
- It was developed for use in medical research as a means of graphically representing a meta-analysis of the results of randomized controlled trials.
- The left-hand column lists the names of the studies (frequently randomized controlled trials or epidemiological studies), commonly in chronological order from the top downwards.
- The right-hand column is a plot of the measure of effect (e.g. an odds ratio) for each of these studies (often represented by a square) incorporating confidence intervals represented by horizontal lines.

Odds Ratio

Odds ratio is an appropriate measure of strength of association for categorical data derived from a case-control study. The odds ratio is often interpreted the same way that relative risk is interpreted when measuring the strength of the association, although this is somewhat controversial when the risk factor being studied is common. It is calculated from the 2x2 table:

	Disease present	Disease absent
Exposed	a	b
Non-exposed	c	d

Odds ratio = ad/bc

Odd ratio interpretation:

- If OR < 1: Negative association (The factor under stay is protective factor).
- If OR = 1: No association
- OR >1: Positive association (The factor under stay is risk factor)

Also, the confidence interval for the Odd's ratio needs to be taken into account.

Interpretation of Significant Odd Ratio is Summarized Below:

Variable	OR	95% confidence index	Comments
Early menarche	1.3	1.2–1.9	Positive, Risk factor, significant
Age <50 yr	0.04	0.01–0.32	Negative, Protective factor, significant
Smoking	0.5	0.02–0.9	Negative Protective factor, significant

Contd...

Contd...

Variable	OR	95% confidence index	Comments
BRCA	1.9	1.1–2.8	Positive, Risk factor, significant
Alcohol	1.0	0.8–1.8	No association
High SES	1.4	0.5–3.5	Sometime it is Positive Risk factor and Sometime it is Negative Risk factor. So it is non-significant risk factor.
Obesity	1.24	1.1–1.7	Positive, Risk factor, significant
No family history	0.3	0.01–0.9	Negative, Protective factor, significant

- Hence, the total number of positive risk factors is three.

Medicine

1. A patient presented to the casualty with right sided hemiparesis and aphasia for a duration of one hour. Mark the following statements as true or false with regards to the management of the patient:

a. rTPA will not be used if CT scan is normal
b. Tenecteplase can be used if CT is normal
c. rTPA will not be used if the patient is on warfarin and the INR is 1.4
d. If CT is normal, thrombolytics need not be used till stroke is confirmed on MRI
e. Tenecteplase should not be used if BP is 160/90 mm Hg

Ans. **a–F, b–T, c–F, d–F, e–F**

Management of Stroke

Administration of IV Recombinant Tissue Plasminogen Activator (rtPA)

Indications

- Clinical diagnosis of stroke
- Onset of symptoms to time of drug administration < 3 hours (can be given till 4.5 hrs if diffusion weighted MRI and perfusion studies are available to evaluate salvageable areas)
- CT scan showing no hemorrhage or edema of > 1/3 of the MCA territory
- Age > 18 years

Contraindications

- Sustained BP >185/110 mm Hg despite treatment
- Platelets <100,000; HCT <25%; glucose <50 or >400 mg/dL
- Use of heparin within 48 hours and prolonged PTT, or elevated INR
- Rapidly improving symptoms
- Prior stroke or head injury within 3 months
- Prior intracranial hemorrhage
- Major surgery in preceding 14 days
- Minor stroke symptoms
- Gastrointestinal bleeding in preceding 21 days
- Recent myocardial infarction
- Coma or stupor

2. Which of the following causes of dementia is associated with visual hallucinations?

a. Lewy body dementia
b. AIDS related dementia
c. Vascular dementia
d. Multisystem atrophy

Ans. **a. Lewy body dementia**

Dementia with Lewy Bodies

Lewy bodies are cytoplasmic inclusions seen in the neurons of the substantia nigra and other pigmented nuclei in patients with Parkinson disease (PD). In recent years, similar neuronal inclusions have been discovered in cortical neurons in patients with dementia. Neurocognitive disorder with Lewy bodies (Lewy body dementia) refers to patients who present with dementia symptoms before or simultaneously with motor disturbances suggestive of PD. Patients with Lewy body disease typically demonstrate fluctuating cognitive impairment, with active confusion and hallucinations, in addition to deterioration of memory and higher cortical functions. This fluctuating, delirium-like presentation distinguishes this disorder from Alzheimer disease. Associated features include early hallucinations, usually visual rather than auditory; mild extrapyramidal signs; or repeated and unexplained falls. Autonomic findings are common, and diffuse Lewy body disease may present as part of the multiple system atrophy or Shy-Drager syndrome. Another associated phenomenon is rapid eye movement (REM) sleep behavior disorder, in which patients act out dreams, shouting, flailing limbs, sometime striking bed partners. This sleep disorder can predate the dementia by decades. The illness progresses at a variable rate to an end stage of severe dementia. Vascular dementias and other physical illness must be excluded.

3. Arrange the following phases of cardiac cycle in sequential order:

a. S1
b. Rapid ejection phase
c. T wave
d. R wave

Ans. d. R wave, a. S1, b. Rapid ejection phase, c. T wave

ECG Waveform

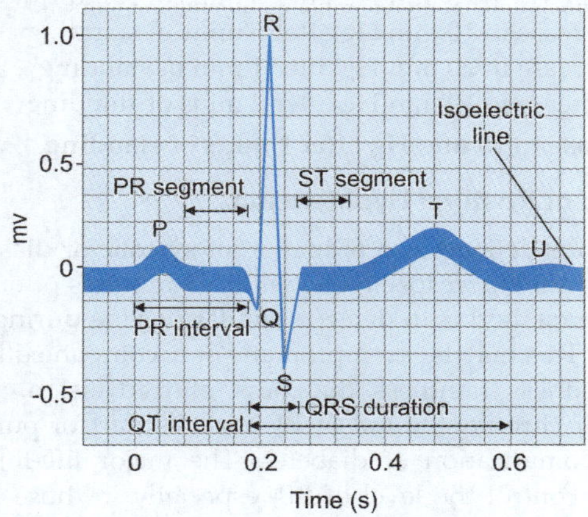

P wave is primarily produced by atrial depolarization, the QRS complex is dominated by ventricular depolarization, and the T wave by ventricular repolarization. The U wave is an inconstant finding that may be due to ventricular myocytes with long action potentials. However, the contributions to this segment are still undetermined.

Relationship between cardiac cycle, ECG and heart sounds has been depicted in the following diagram:

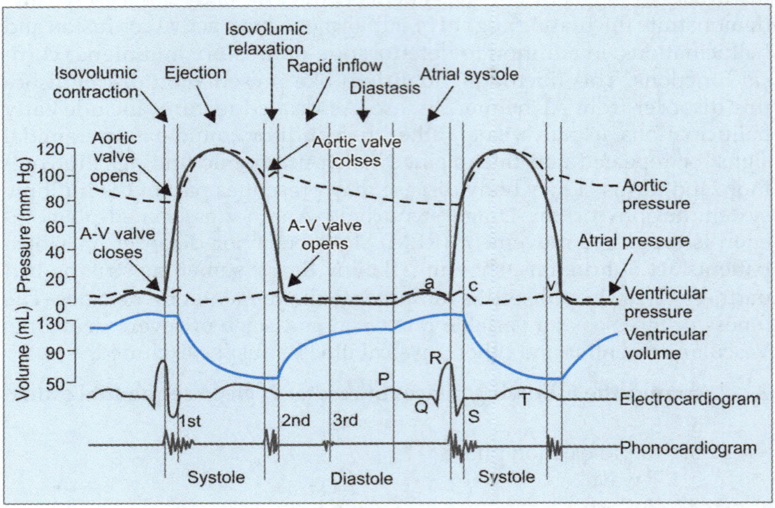

4. Which of the following is defined as postural hypotension?

a. Decrease in 20 mm Hg after 3 mins of standing
b. Decrease in 10 mm Hg after 5 mins of standing
c. Decrease in 20 mm Hg after 1 min of standing
d. Decrease in 10 mm Hg after 2 mins of standing

Ans. **a. Decrease in 20 mm Hg after 3 mins of standing**

Orthostatic or Postural Hypotension

This condition is defined as a reduction of systolic or diastolic BP of at least 20 or 10 mm Hg, respectively, within 3 minutes of quiet standing. An alternative method is to detect a similar decline during head-up tilt at 60 degrees. This may be asymptomatic or accompanied by symptoms of light-headedness, faintness, dizziness, blurred vision, and cognitive impairment. If chronic, the fall of BP may be part of pure autonomic failure or a complication of diabetes. The major life-limiting failure is inability to control the level of BP, especially in those patients with orthostatic hypotension who concomitantly have supine hypertension. In these patients, there are great and swift changes in pressure so that the patients faint as a result of profound hypotension on standing and have very severe hypertension when supine. Often the heart rate is fixed as well. The supine hypertensive person is subject to serious consequences, such as left ventricular hypertrophy and stroke.

5. Which of the following statements is not a contraindication for thrombolysis in DVT?

a. INR > 1.4
b. Suspected aortic dissection
c. Prior intracranial hemorrhage
d. Craniofacial trauma within the last 3 months

Ans. a. INR > 1.4

Contraindications to fibrinolytic therapy for deep venous thrombosis or acute pulmonary embolism.

Absolute Contraindications

- Prior intracranial hemorrhage
- Known structural cerebral vascular lesion
- Known malignant intracranial neoplasm
- Ischemic stroke within three months (excluding stroke within three hours)
- Suspected aortic dissection
- Active bleeding or bleeding diathesis (excluding menses)
- Significant closed-head trauma or facial trauma within three months

Relative Contraindications

- History of chronic, severe, poorly controlled hypertension
- Severe uncontrolled hypertension on presentation (SBP >180 mm Hg or DBP >110 mm Hg)
- History of ischemic stroke more than three months prior
- Traumatic or prolonged (>10 minute) CPR or major surgery less than three weeks
- Recent (within two to four weeks) internal bleeding
- Noncompressible vascular punctures
- Recent invasive procedure
- For streptokinase/anistreplase—Prior exposure (more than five days ago) or prior allergic reaction to these agents
- Pregnancy
- Active peptic ulcer
- Pericarditis or pericardial fluid
- Current use of anticoagulant (e.g., warfarin sodium) that has produced an elevated international normalized ratio (INR) >1.7 or prothrombin time (PT) >15 seconds

- Age >75 years
- Diabetic retinopathy

6. Calculate the anion gap- Na^+– 137 mEq/L, K^+ – 3 mEq/L, Ca^{2+} – 5 mEq/L, PO_4^{3-} –3 mEq/L, HCO_3^- – 15 mEq/L, Cl^- – 110 mEq/L:

a. 15
b. 12
c. 17
d. 10

Ans. b. 12

The anion gap (AG) represents the concentration of all the unmeasured anions in the plasma. The normal value for the serum anion gap is 8–16 mEq/L.

Anion Gap: Na^- (Cl^+ HCO_3^-) = 137– (110 + 15) = 12
Causes of high-anion gap metabolic acidosis

Lactic Acidosis

Toxins

- Ethylene glycol
- Methanol
- Salicylates
- Propylene glycol
- Pyroglutamic acid (5-oxoproline)

Ketoacidosis

- Diabetic
- Alcoholic
- Starvation

Renal Failure (Acute and Chronic)

Causes of non–anion gap acidosis

- Gastrointestinal bicarbonate loss
  - Diarrhea
  - External pancreatic or small-bowel drainage
  - Ureterosigmoidostomy, jejunal loop, ileal loop
  - Drugs
    - Calcium chloride (acidifying agent)
    - Magnesium sulfate (diarrhea)
    - Cholestyramine (bile acid diarrhea)
- Renal acidosis
  - Hypokalemia
    - Proximal RTA (type 2)

Drug-induced: acetazolamide, topiramate

- ❖ Distal (classic) RTA (type 1)

  Drug induced: amphotericin B, ifosfamide

- ❑ Hyperkalemia
  - ❖ Generalized distal nephron dysfunction (type 4 RTA)
    - Mineralocorticoid deficiency
    - Mineralocorticoid resistance (PHA I, autosomal dominant)
    - Voltage defect (PHA I, autosomal recessive, and PHA II)
    - Tubulointerstitial disease
- ❑ Normokalemia
  - ❖ Chronic progressive kidney disease

7. Which of the following is not a component of qSOFA score?

a. Glasgow coma score <15
b. Respiratory rate >22 per min
c. Systolic BP <100 mm Hg
d. Absent pupillary light reflex

Ans. d. Absent pupillary light reflex

The qSOFA score (also known as quickSOFA) is a bedside prompt that may identify patients with suspected infection who are at greater risk for a poor outcome outside the intensive care unit (ICU). It uses three criteria, assigning one point each for low blood pressure (SBP ≤100 mm Hg), high respiratory rate (≥ 22 breaths per min), or altered mentation (Glasgow coma scale < 15). The score ranges from 0 to 3 points. The presence of 2 or more qSOFA points near the onset of infection was associated with a greater risk of death or prolonged intensive care unit stay. These are outcomes that are more common in infected patients who may be septic than those with uncomplicated infection. Based upon these findings, the Third International Consensus Definitions for Sepsis recommends qSOFA as a simple prompt to identify infected patients outside the ICU who are likely to be septic.

8. A patient was exposed to hepatitis B infection. Which of the following markers will always be present irrespective of whether the patient recovers from the infection or not?

a. HbsAg
b. Anti Hbs
c. Anti Hbc
d. HbeAg

Ans. c. Anti Hbc

Various serologic patterns of hepatitis B infection					
HBsAg	***Anti-HBs***	***Anti-HBc***	***HBeAg***	***Anti-HBe***	***Interpretation***
+	–	IgM	+	–	➤ Acute hepatitis B, high infectivity
+	–	IgM	+	–	➤ Chronic hepatitis B, high infectivity
+	–	IgM	–	+	➤ Late acute or chronic hepatitis B, low infectivity ➤ HBeAg-negative ('precore—mutant') hepatitis B (chronic or rarely acute)
+	+	+	+/–	+/–	➤ HbsAg of one subtype and heterotypic anti-Hbs (common) ➤ Process of seroconversion from HbsAg to anti Hbs (rare)
–	–	IgM	+/–	+/–	➤ Acute hepatitis B ➤ Window period for anti-HbsAg
–	–	IgM	–	+/–	➤ Low-level hepatitis B carrier ➤ Hepatitis B in remote past
–	+	IgM	–	+/–	➤ Recovery from hepatitis B
–	+	–	–	–	➤ Immunization with HbsAg (after vaccination) ➤ Hepatitis B in the remote past ➤ False-positive

9. Bone mineral density screening is recommended after the age of:

a. 55 years
b. 50 years
c. 60 years
d. 65 years

Ans. **d. 65 years**

Bone Mineral Density Screening

The biggest risk factor for developing osteoporosis is increasing age. Although many women expect to be screened around the time of menopause, routine BMD screening is not recommended until the age of 65. The National Osteoporosis Foundation recommends screening all women aged 65 and older and screening younger postmenopausal women if there is a concern based on their risk-factor profile. The USPSTF recommends screening women aged 65 and older and only screening younger women whose fracture risk is equal to or greater than that of a 65-year-old white woman who has no additional risk factors. The FRAX tool can be used to calculate 10-year risk of osteoporotic fracture. Most guidelines do not specifically address how often a woman should undergo BMD testing. However, decisions about when to rescreen should probably be based on the results of initial screening. Women with normal BMD or mild osteopenia at baseline can be screened less often than women who are near the threshold for osteoporosis. Treatment is generally recommended in women who have a T score below –2.5, who have already had a fracture or who have a T score in the osteopenic range but are at high risk for fracture.

10. The given pattern of EEG found in:

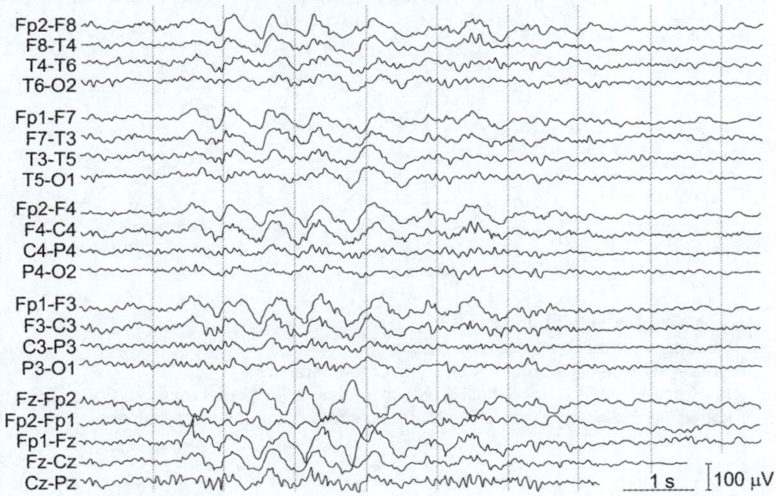

a. Hepatic encephalopathy
b. Creutzfeldt-Jakob disease
c. GTCS
d. Herpes simplex encephalitis

Ans. **b. Creutzfeldt-Jakob disease**

Creutzfeldt-Jakob Disease (CJD)

- CJD is caused by prions, transmissible protein particles.
- CJD patient is younger than in Alzheimer.
- Rapidly progressive dementia and the presence of myoclonus are most common manifestation.
- Although the EEG is abnormal, the most accurate diagnostic test is a brain biopsy.
- *Pathological Findings*: PrPSC deposition, panlaminar spongiosis
- CSF shows a 14-3-3 protein. The presence of the 14-3-3 protein spares the patient the need for brain biopsy.

Abnormal Waveforms in EEG

Hepatic encephalopathy

- Triphasic waves

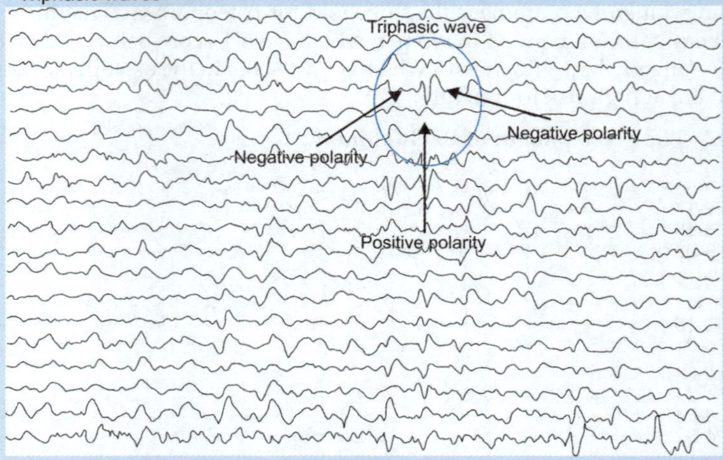

Herpes simplex encephalitis

- Periodic lateralized epileptiform discharge.
- Notice the repetitive burst of activity over temporal area.
- In Herpes simplex encephalitis, which mainly affects the temporal lobe, EEG shows Periodic lateralized epileptiform discharge over the temporal lobe.

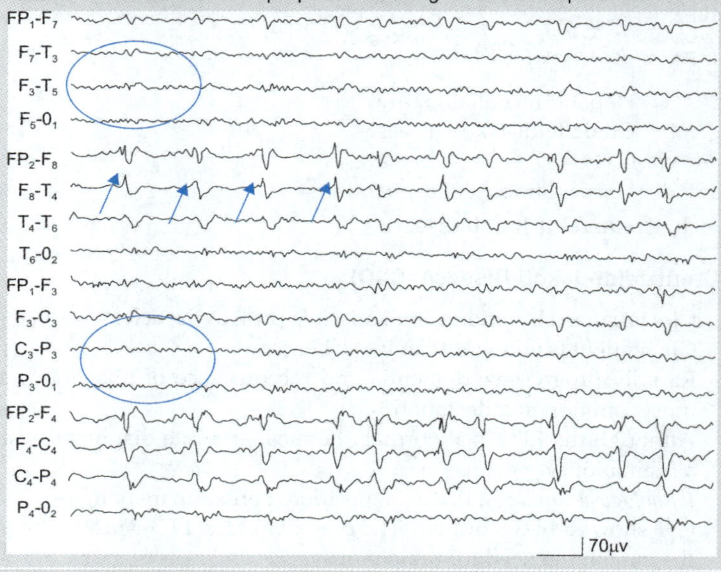

GTCS

- Generalized repetitive sharp activity with synchronicity in all leads.

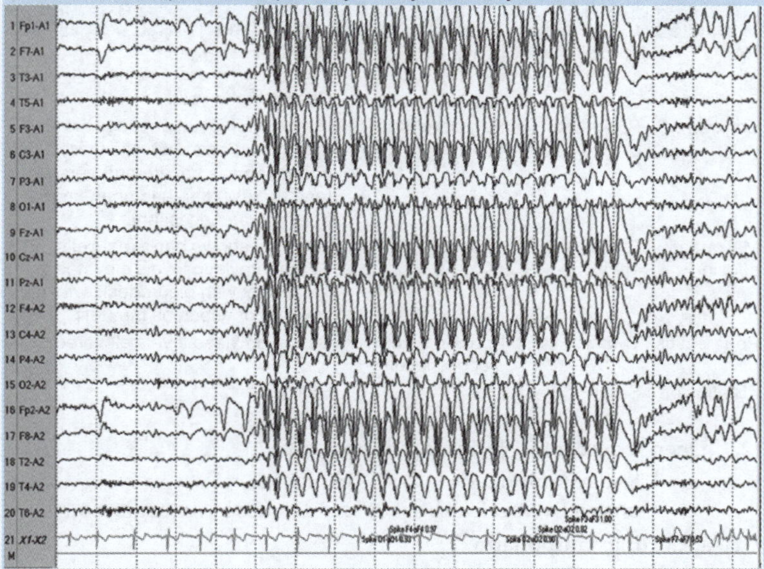

11. All of the following characteristics are found in pleural effusion fluid of a Rheumatoid Arthritis patient; *except*:

a. RA factor positive
b. High glucose
c. Cholesterol crystals
d. High LDH

Ans. b. High glucose

Types of Pleural Effusion

	Transudative	Exudative
Definition	This condition is due to imbalance of pressure between hydrostatic pressure and oncotic pressure	This condition results from inflammation
Causes	➢ CHF is most common cause ➢ Nephrotic syndrome ➢ Liver disease ➢ Pulmonary embolism ➢ Atelectasis	➢ Parapneumonic effusions (pneumonia)—MC ➢ Malignancy (Lung (36%) > breast (25%) > lymphoma (10%) ➢ Tuberculosis ➢ Pulmonary embolism ➢ Collagen vascular disease (Rheumatoid arthritis, systemic lupus erythematosus) ➢ Drug induced ➢ Pancreatitis

Characteristics of Various Exudative Pleural Effusions

Type	Gross appearance	Glucose	Others
RA	Turbid greenish	Low (<60% mg%)	➢ High LDH ➢ RA Factor: +ve ➢ Cholesterol crystal
Empyema	Pus in the pleural space	Polymorphs	➢ Needs intercostal drainage (via thoracentesis) and antibiotic therapy ➢ If empyema is severe and persistent, rib resection and open drainage may be necessary
Malignant effusion	Bloody effusion	<60 mg%	➢ Cytology shows abnormal cells ➢ Serum amylase levels elevated ➢ Treatment with pleurodesis with doxycycline or asbestos free talc
Pancreatitis	Turbid	Equal to serum glucose levels	➢ Serum amylase levels elevated
TB effusion	Serous	Low	➢ High protein

12. Deep y descent in JVP is seen in all *except*:

a. Cardiac tamponade b. RCM
c. Constrictive pericarditis d. Tricuspid regurgitation

Ans. a. Cardiac tamponade

Jugular Venous Pulse

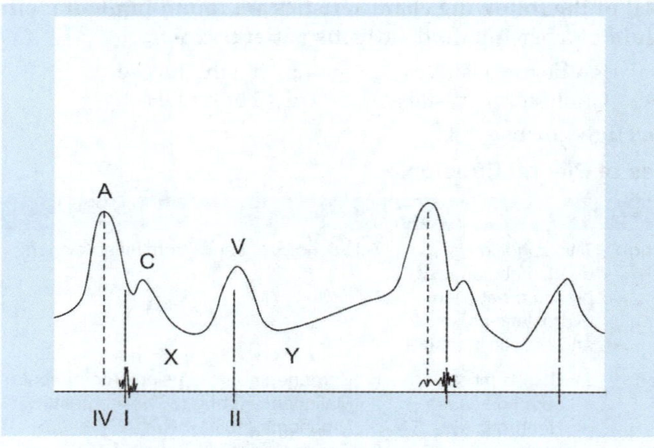

- A wave represents right atrial presystolic contraction and occurs just after the electrocardiographic P wave and just before the first heart sound (I).
- The C wave may reflect the carotid pulsation in the neck and/or an early systolic increase in right atrial pressure as the right ventricle

pushes the closed tricuspid valve into the right atrium. (Isovolumetric contraction).

- The X descent follows the A wave just as atrial pressure continues to fall. (Atrial relaxation).
- The V wave represents atrial filling during ventricular systole and peaks at the second heart sound (II).
- The Y descent corresponds to the fall in right atrial pressure after tricuspid valve opening. (Diastolic ventricular filling).

Various abnormalities in JVP are summarized below:

Elevated "A" wave	Cannon "A" wave
➢ Tricuspid stenosis ➢ Decreased ventricular compliance due to ventricular failure, pulmonic valve stenosis, or pulmonary hypertension	➢ Complete heart block ➢ Premature ventricular contraction ➢ During ventricular tachycardia, ventricular pacing ➢ During junctional rhythm and tachycardia
Absent "A" wave	**Elevated "V" wave**
➢ Atrial fibrillation or atrial standstill.	➢ Right ventricular failure ➢ Tricuspid regurgitation ➢ Restrictive cardiomyopathy (Reduced atrial compliance)
"A" wave equal to "V" wave	**Prominent "X" descent**
➢ Hypervolemia ➢ Cardiac tamponade ➢ Atrial septal defect ➢ Constrictive pericarditis	➢ Right ventricular ischemia with preservation of atrial contractility ➢ Cardiac tamponade ➢ Atrial septal defect ➢ Subacute constriction and possibly chronic constriction
Prominent "Y" descent	**Blunted "X" descent**
➢ Tricuspid regurgitation ➢ Constrictive pericarditis ➢ Atrial septal defect ➢ Restrictive cardiomyopathies	➢ Atrial fibrillation ➢ Tricuspid regurgitation ➢ Right atrial ischemia
Blunted "Y" descent	**Elevated jugular venous pressure**
➢ Right atrial myxoma ➢ Cardiac tamponade ➢ Tricuspid stenosis ➢ Right ventricular ischemia	➢ Pericardial effusion with tamponade physiology ➢ Right ventricular failure ➢ Superior vena caval obstruction ➢ Intravascular volume overload conditions due to valvular disease (tricuspid or pulmonic stenosis or regurgitation), right ventricular ischemia or infarction, cardiomyopathy or secondary to left heart failure (mitral stenosis/regurgitation, aortic stenosis/regurgitation, cardiomyopathy, myocardial ischemia/ infarction) ➢ Obstructive atrial myxoma ➢ Constrictive pericarditis

13. A patient had recurrent optic neuritis of both eyes with Extensive Transverse Myelitis. Visual acuity in Right eye is 6/60 and visual acuity in Left eye 6/18. Patient showed 50% response to steroids. Diagnosis is:

a. NMO (Neuromyelitis optica)
b. SACD (Subacute combined degeneration of spinal cord)
c. Posterior cerebral artery stroke
d. Neurosyphilis

Ans. **a. NMO**

Diagnostic Criteria for Neuromyelitis Optica (NMO)

- Required:
  - Optic neuritis
  - Acute transverse myelitis
- Supportive (2 of 3 criteria required):
  - Longitudinally extensive cord lesion extending over 3 or more vertebral segments
  - Brain magnetic resonance imaging normal or not meeting criteria for Multiple Sclerosis
  - Aquaporin-4 seropositivity
- 'Cloud-like' appearance sometimes seen in MRI, but unlike to MS
- *CSF Findings*: Pleocytosis, neutrophils and eosinophils
- *Next investigation will be*: Anti NMO IgG (in blood > CSF)
- *Best treatment*: Steroids + IV Ig

Subacute Combined Degeneration of Spinal Cord

- Loss of reflexes due to an associated peripheral neuropathy.
- Diagnostic clue: Babinski sign.
- Optic atrophy and irritability seen in advanced cases.
- *Lab findings*: Macrocytic red blood cell, low serum B12 concentration, elevated serum homocysteine.
- *Best investigation*: Anti-parietal cell antibodies and Schilling test.
- *Treatment*: Vitamin B12 therapy (1000 μg given intramuscular at regular intervals).

Neurosyphilis

- *Neurological involvement*: Argyll-Robertson pupil, Tabes dorsalis, general paresis, rarely a gumma or aortitis.
- Initial diagnostic test:
  - Lumbar puncture for neurosyphilis
    - FTA is 100% sensitive in CSF
    - CSF VDRL is only 50% sensitive.
- *Treatment*: IV penicillin. Desensitize if penicillin-allergic.

14. Which of the following most associated with respiratory alkalosis?

a. Assisted control mode ventilation
b. Controlled mandatory
c. Pressure controlled
d. SIMV

Ans. a. Assisted control mode ventilation

Modes of Ventilation

Volume Modes

Assist-Control Ventilation (ACV)

Also known as continuous mandatory ventilation (CMV). Each breath is either an assist or control breath, but they are all of the same volume. The larger the volume, the more expiratory time required. If the I:E ratio is less than 1:2, progressive hyperinflation may result. ACV is particularly undesirable for patients who breathe rapidly-they may induce both hyperinflation and respiratory alkalosis. Note that mechanical ventilation does not eliminate the work of breathing, because the diaphragm may still be very active.

Synchronized Intermittent-Mandatory Ventilation (SIMV)

Guarantees a certain number of breaths, but unlike ACV, patient breaths are partially their own, reducing the risk of hyperinflation or alkalosis. Mandatory breaths are synchronized to coincide with spontaneous respirations. Disadvantages of SIMV are increased work of breathing and a tendency to reduce cardiac output, which may prolong ventilator dependency. The addition of pressure support on top of spontaneous breaths can reduce some of the work of breathing. SIMV has been shown to decrease cardiac output in patients with left-ventricular dysfunction.

Pressure Modes

Pressure-Controlled Ventilation (PCV)

Less risk of barotrauma as compared to ACV and SIMV. Does not allow for patient-initiated breaths. The inspiratory flow pattern decreases exponentially, reducing peak pressures and improving gas exchange. The major disadvantage is that there are no guarantees for volume, especially when lung mechanics are changing. Thus, PCV has traditionally been preferred for patients with neuromuscular disease but otherwise normal lungs.

Pressure Support Ventilation (PSV)

Allows the patient to determine inflation volume and respiratory frequency (but not pressure, as this is pressure-controlled), thus can only be used to augment spontaneous breathing. Pressure support can be used to overcome the resistance of ventilator tubing in another cycle (5–10 cm

H_2O are generally used, especially during weaning), or to augment spontaneous breathing. PSV can be delivered through specialized face masks.

15. Tigroid appearance of white matter on MRI is seen in:

a. Pantothenate kinase deficiency
b. Pelizaeus-Merzbacher disease
c. Neuroferritinopathy
d. Aceruloplasminemia

Ans. b. Pelizaeus-Merzbacher disease

- The Tigroid pattern or stripe sign is also known as leopard skin sign results from dark-spots or stripes (spared perivascular white matter) within bright demyelinated periventricular white matter on T2W images.
- It is most commonly seen in:
  - Peizaeus-Merzbacher disease (PMD)
    - The human neural stem cells have both neurogenic and gliogenic potential, and when delivered to white matter regions in experimental animals most persisting cells had become oligodendrocytes. This supported use of the cells to promote myelin formation in conditions such as PMD.
  - Metachromatic leukodystrophy
  - Autosomal recessive spastic ataxia of Charlevoix

16. A patient presents with recent onset breathlessness and ECG is taken. ECG is shown below. What is the diagnosis?

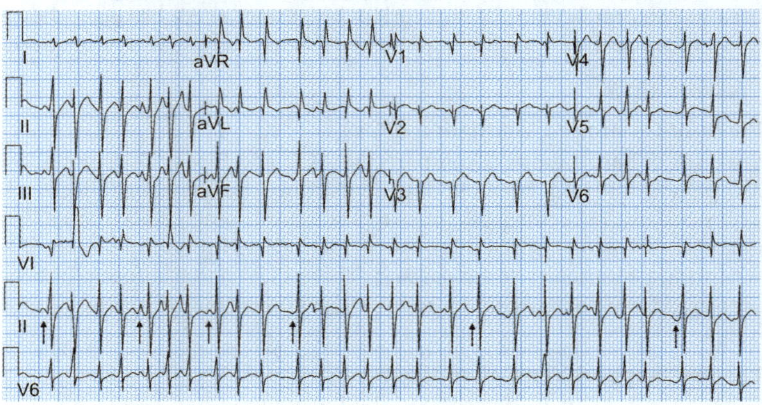

a. AF
b. PSVT
c. AMI
d. MAT

Ans. d. MAT

Rhythm Abnormalities on ECG

Junctional Rhythm

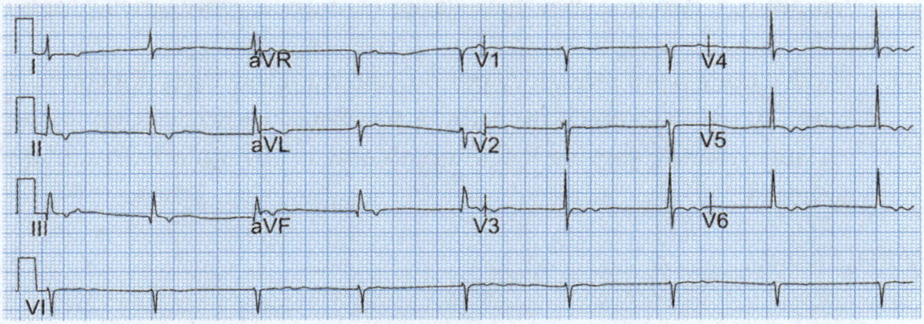

- The QRS complex is narrow, with a rate typically between 40 and 60 bpm.
- P waves are absent, retrograde, very slow, or unrelated to the QRS complex.

Ventricular Rhythm

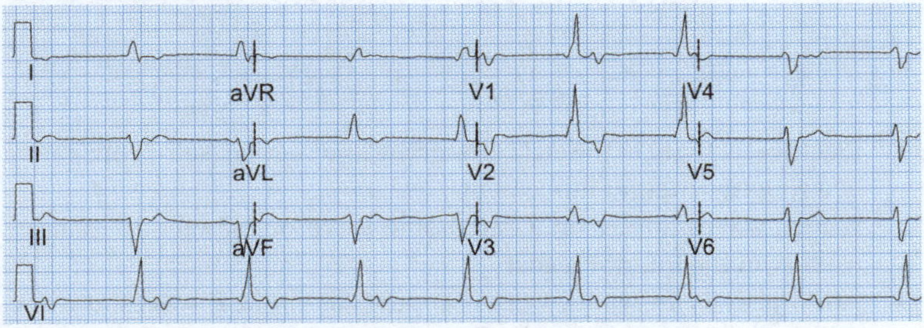

- The QRS complex is wider than 120 ms, with a rate typically between 20 and 40 bpm.
- The T wave is discordant relative to the QRS.

Atrial Fibrillation

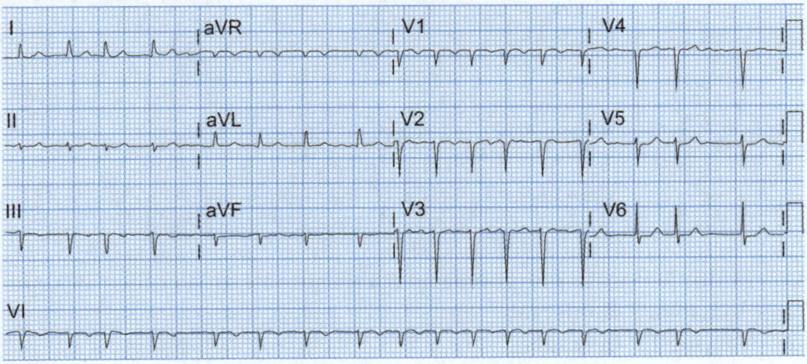

- Electrical activity in the atria is chaotic. The ECG baseline, representing the ongoing chaotic atrial activity, is unorganized. The resulting "rumbling" baseline may have large or indiscernibly small ampli0 tude.
- The AV node has a refractory period, and therefore does not conduct every signal it receives from the atria. Thus, ventricles depolarize variably creating varying R-R intervals and an "irregularly irregular" pattern.

Atrial Flutter

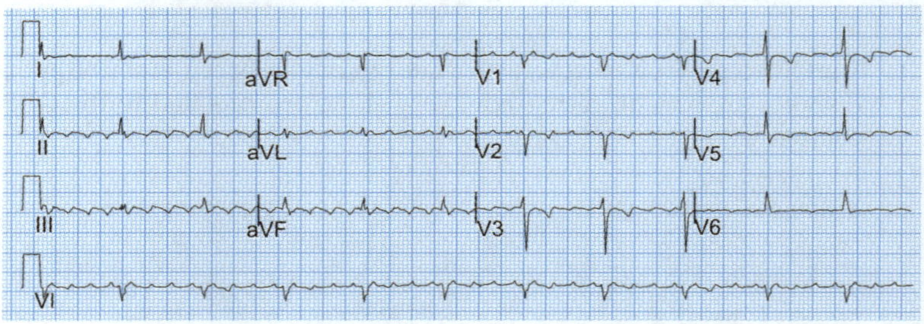

- Electrical activity in the atria is ongoing and regular, self-propagating in a roughly circular movement.
- Flutter waves appear in a rapid sine wave or "sawtooth" pattern, usually in the inferior leads.
- Atrial activity in lead V1 often appears as rapid P waves at a rate approximating 300 bpm.

Multifocal Atrial Tachycardia

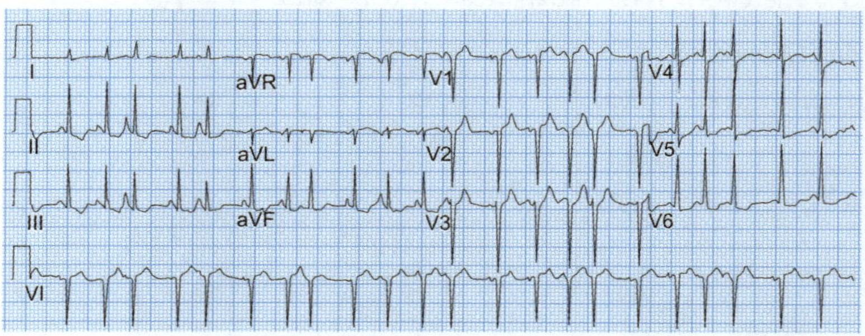

- Multiple P-wave morphologies with heart rate greater than 100 bpm
- A chaotic R-R interval
- Varying PR intervals

Ventricular Tachycardia

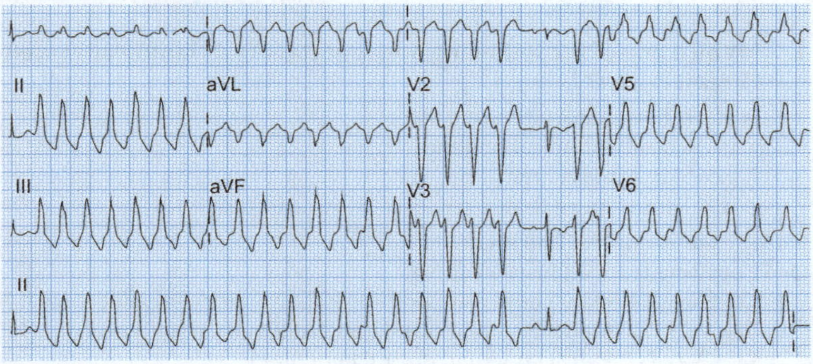

- Tachycardia (usually >120 bpm) with a wide QRS complex.
- AV dissociation is present; P waves may appear periodically in the T wave or baseline.
- "Capture" beats may occur if atrial depolarization occurs prior to the intrinsic firing of the ventricle.
- "Fusion" beats may occur if atrial depolarization passes through the AV node at the same time as the intrinsic ventricle depolarization, producing a QRS that appears to be different or narrower than the other VT QRS complexes.

Ventricular Flutter

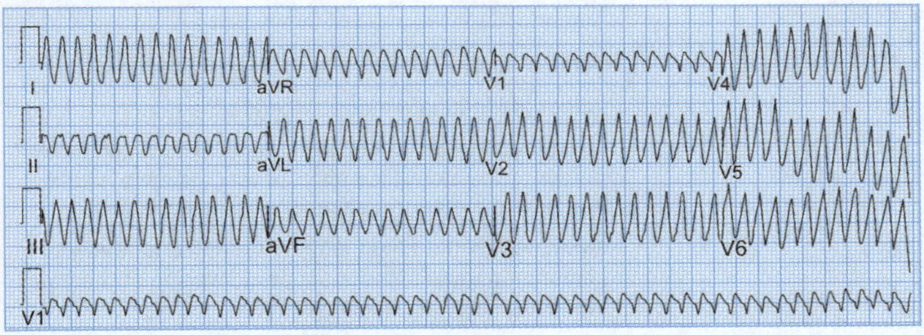

- Tachycardia with a wide monomorphic QRS complex.
- Ventricular rate may be very rapid (300 bpm).
- Sine wave appearance with regular large oscillations.

Surgery

1. Which one of the following does not classify as locally advanced breast cancer?

a. Inflammatory breast cancer
b. Chest wall involvement
c. Skin involvement
d. Tumor more than 4 cm

Ans. d. Tumor more than 4 cm

- Locally advanced breast cancer
  - Any T4 (skin, chest wall, both or inflammatory breast cancer)
  - Any N2 (matted lymph nodes or internal mammary lymph nodes)
  - Any N3 (infraclavicular, supraclavicular)
  - With M0

TNM Staging of Breast Cancer

T0	No evidence of primary tumor
Tis (DCIS)*	Ductal carcinoma *in situ*
Tis (Paget)	Paget disease of the nipple NOT associated with invasive carcinoma and/or carcinoma *in situ* (DCIS) in the underlying breast parenchyma. Carcinomas in the breast parenchyma associated with Paget disease are categorized based on the size and characteristics of the parenchymal disease, although the presence of Paget disease should still be noted.
T1	Tumor ≤20 mm in greatest dimension
T2	Tumor >20 mm but ≤50 mm in greatest dimension
T3	Tumor >50 mm in greatest dimension
T4	Tumor of any size with direct extension to the chest wall and/or to the skin (ulceration or macroscopic nodules); invasion of the dermis alone does not qualify as T4
T4a	Extension to the chest wall; invasion or adherence to pectoralis muscle in the absence of invasion of chest wall structures does not qualify as T4
T4b	Ulceration and/or ipsilateral macroscopic satellite nodules and/or edema (including peau d'orange) of the skin that does not meet the criteria for inflammatory carcinoma
T4c	Both T4a and T4b are present
T4d	Inflammatory carcinoma

***Note:** Lobular carcinoma *in situ* (LCIS) is a benign entity and is removed from TNM staging in the *AJCC Cancer Staging Manual, 8th edition*.

Contd...

Contd...

	Regional lymph nodes—Clinical (N)
cN0	No regional lymph node metastases (by imaging or clinical examination)
cN1	Metastases to movable ipsilateral Level I, II axillary lymph node(s)
cN2	
cN2a	Metastases in ipsilateral Level I, II axillary lymph nodes fixed to one another (matted) or to other structures
cN2b	Metastases only in ipsilateral internal mammary nodes in the absence of axillary lymph node metastases
cN3	
cN3a	Metastases in ipsilateral infraclavicular lymph node(s)
cN3b	Metastases in ipsilateral internal mammary lymph node(s) and axillary lymph node(s)
cN3c	Metastases in ipsilateral supraclavicular lymph node

2. Percentage of SSI rate in patients with a clean contaminated wound?

a. <10%
b. 1–2%
c. 10–20%
d. 20–30%

Ans. a. <10%

Classification of wounds and their infection rates are given below:

- *Clean wound*: An incision in which no inflammation is encountered in a surgical procedure, without a break in sterile technique, and during which the respiratory, alimentary and genitourinary tracts are not entered- 1–2%.
- *Clean contaminated*: An incision through which the respiratory, alimentary or genitourinary tract is entered under controlled conditions but with no contamination encountered- 7–10% (without antibiotic prophylaxis); 4–5 (with antibiotic prophylaxis)
- *Contaminated*: An incision undertaken during an operation in which there is a major break in sterile technique or gross spillage from the gastrointestinal tract, or an incision in which acute, non-purulent inflammation is encountered. Open traumatic wounds that are more than 12–24 hours old also fall into this category- 10–20% (without); 7-8% (with prophylaxis)
- *Dirty*: An incision undertaken during an operation in which the viscera are perforated or when acute inflammation with pus is encountered during the operation (for example, emergency surgery for faecal

peritonitis), and for traumatic wounds where treatment is delayed, and there is faecal contamination or devitalized tissue present->20% (without); 8-10% (with antibiotics).

3. Which of the following scoring systems is used for grading wound infections?

a. Southampton score
b. ASA score
c. SIRS score
d. Glasgow score

Ans. a. Southampton score

Southampton Wound Grading System

Grade/appearance	Subtype/Appearance
0: Normal healing	
I: Normal healing with mild bruising or erythema	Ia: Some bruising Ib: Considerable bruising Ic: Mild erythema
II: Erythema plus other signs of inflammations	IIa: At one point IIb: Around sutures IIc: Along wound
III: Clear or hemoserous discharge	IIIa: At one point only (<2 cm) IIIb: Along wound (>2 cm) IIIc: Large volume IIId: Prolonged (>3 days)
IV: Pus	IVa: At one point only (<2 cm) IVb: Along wound (>2 cm)
V: Deep or severe wound infection with or without tissue breakdown; Hematoma requiring aspiration	

4. Which of the following is not a topical hemostatic agent?

a. Kaolin
b. Zeolite
c. Boric acid
d. Chitosan

Ans. c. Boric acid

Topical Hemostatic Agents

Topical hemostatic agents can play an important role in helping to facilitate surgical hemostasis. These agents are classified based on their mechanism of action, and many act at specific stages in the coagulation cascade and take advantage of natural physiologic responses to bleeding. The ideal topical hemostatic agent has significant hemostatic action, minimal tissue reactivity, nonantigenicity, in vivo biodegradability, ease of sterilization, low cost, and can be tailored to specific needs.

Absorbable agents include gelatin foams (Gelfoam), oxidized cellulose (Surgicel), and microfibrillar collagens (Avitene). Both gelatin foam and oxidized cellulose provide a physical matrix for clotting initiation, while microfibrillar collagens facilitate platelet adherence and activation. Biologic agents include topical thrombin, fibrin sealants (FloSeal), and platelet sealants (Vitagel). Human or recombinant thrombin derivatives, which facilitate the formation of fibrin clots and subsequent activation of several clotting factors, take advantage of natural physiologic processes, thereby avoiding foreign body or inflammatory reactions.

Structural composition of the most commonly used hemostatic agents:

QuikClot, a manufactured granular mineral zeolite, is composed of oxides of silicon, sodium, aluminium and magnesium. It also includes small amounts of quartz. This agent acts as a molecular sieve and rapidly adsorbs water. It holds the water molecules in pores, by hydrogen bonds, through a nonchemical, physical reaction.

The self-expanding hemostatic polymer is formed from an absorbent material, which is composed of a superabsorbent polymer and a wicking binder. The self-expanding hemostatic polymer acts through two mechanisms to control hemorrhage, as follows: (1) *mechanical*: rapid swelling of SEHP following blood absorption results in exertion of a direct tamponade effect on the wound surface and (2) *biochemical*: concentration of coagulation factors and platelets following absorption of the aqueous phase of blood at the site of bleeding, leading to promotion of the clotting cascade.

Celox is an entirely biocompatible and biodegradable substance, a chitosan (a mucoadhesive component that maintains the silica in contact with the wound) granule that promotes clot formation through adsorption and dehydration, and the advancement of red blood cell bonding.

The mRDH is a biocompatible material and is composed of poly-N-acetyl glucosamine (pGlcNAc) nanofiber material. mRDH causes vasoconstriction, platelet activation and red blood cell aggregation.

TraumaStat is composed of chitosan, silica (a strong activator of the intrinsic clotting cascade) and polyethylene, which forms the primary structure of the dressing. The Trauma Stat dressing is conformable, similar to gauze, and covers a much greater surface area than is currently possible with other chitosan dressings or gauzes.

The Hem Con bandage is a lyophilized chitosan derivative, working through the attraction of the protonated amine groups on chitosan molecules to the negatively charged residues on red blood cell membranes, together with the adsorption of chitosan for fibrinogen and plasma proteins.

Wound Stat is composed of smectite granules, and is considered to stop bleeding by means of the granules that absorb water, swelling and forming a clay substance with high plasticity that adheres to the tissue and seals the sites of hemorrhage.

5. Arrange the following in the correct order of removing PPE after surgery?

a. Goggles
b. Mask
c. Gloves
d. Gown

Ans. **c. Gloves, a. Goggles, d. Gown, b. Mask**

Sequence for removing PPE

1. Gloves
2. Face shield or goggles
3. Gown
4. Mask or respirator

The sequence for removing PPE is intended to limit opportunities for self-contamination. The gloves are considered the most contaminated pieces of PPE and are therefore removed first. The face shield or goggles are next because they are more cumbersome and would interfere with removal of other PPEs. The gown is third in the sequence, followed by the mask or respirator.

6. All are features of SIRS *except*:

a. RR > 24 and $PaCO_2$ < 22 mm Hg
b. WBC counts >11000 or <4000 per microlitre
c. Temp <36 and >38 degrees C
d. PR >90 per min

Ans. **a. RR > 24 and $PaCO_2$ < 22 mm Hg**

Systemic inflammatory response syndrome (SIRS)

Defined as a systemic response to a nonspecific infectious or noninfectious insult—such as from burns, pancreatitis, an autoimmune disorder, ischemia, or trauma—the presence of two or more of the following clinical criteria help establish the diagnosis of SIRS:

1. Body temperature higher than 38°C (100.4°F) or lower than 36°C (96.8°F),
2. Heart rate faster than 90 beats per minute,
3. Respiratory rate more than 20 breaths per minute or hyperventilation with an arterial carbon dioxide tension ($PaCO_2$) less than 32 mm Hg, or
4. Abnormal white blood cell count (greater than 12,000/mcL or less than 4000/mcL or greater than 10% immature [band] forms).

When a source of infection is confirmed, SIRS is categorized as sepsis. The consensus group that issued the 2016 definition of sepsis recommended eliminating the term SIRS. However, this remains controversial in the absence of strong evidence to suggest that SIRS criteria are an inferior way to identify patients at risk for sepsis. Studies on the impact of the new sepsis definitions (SEPSIS-3) as a predictive measure of mortality are ongoing.

7. Most common mediastinal tumor?

a. Thymoma
b. Neurogenic
c. Lymphoma
d. Bronchial cyst

Ans. a. Thymoma

- Thymoma is the most common mediastinal mass
- Neurogenic tumors are most common in the posterior mediastinum in children.

Superior mediastinum	Anterior mediastinum	Posterior mediastinum	Middle mediastinum
➤ Lymphoma ➤ Thymoma ➤ Thyroid lesions ➤ Metastatic carcinoma ➤ Parathyroid tumors	➤ Thymoma (MC) ➤ Teratoma ➤ Lymphoma ➤ Thyroid lesions ➤ Parathyroid tumors	➤ Neurogenic tumors (MC) (schwannoma, neurofibroma) ➤ Lymphoma ➤ Gastroenteric hernia	➤ Bronchogenic cyst ➤ Pericardial cyst ➤ Lymphoma

8. A male came to the ER after car accident. He had dyspnea and chest pain with ecchymosis on anterior chest wall. On examination, pulse -120/min, BP-80/50 mm Hg. Breaths sounds were decreased on left side, JVP was raised and tympanic note was present on percussion. Pelvis and extremities were normal. What is the next immediate step in the management?

a. Intubate the patient
b. Needle insertion in 5th ICS
c. Urgent fluid infusion
d. Chest X-ray

Ans. b. Needle insertion in 5th ICS

Tension Pneumothorax

- It develops when air flows into the thoracic cavity through a one-way valve mechanism, resulting in collapse of the affected lung.

Clinical features:

- It is essentially a clinical diagnosis.
- Patient presents with sudden onset dyspnea and distended neck veins
- Mediastinal shift to the opposite side with tracheal deviation, hyperresonance & absent breath sounds over the affected hemithorax.

Treatment:

- Treatment consists of immediate decompression by rapid insertion of a large-bore needle into 4th or 5th intercostal space in the mid-clavicular line of the affected hemithorax.

- This is immediately followed by insertion of a chest tube through the 5th intercostal space in anterior axillary line.

9. True about inflammatory aneurysm:

a. Surgical management is the treatment of choice for large aneurysms
b. Bifurcation of ICA is the most common site
c. They are pseudoaneurysms
d. Smoking is not a risk factor

Ans. **a. Surgical management is the treatment of choice for large aneurysms**

Inflammatory aneurysms are degenerative aneurysms that elicit a unique inflammatory response adjacent to the external calcified layer of the aneurysm wall. Although similar to retroperitoneal fibrosis, the inflammation is usually confined to the anterior aorta and iliac arteries. Male sex, smoking and a genetic predisposition, are the main risk factors. The percentage of patients with inflammatory abdominal aortic aneurysm who smoke is high, ranging from 77% to 100% of patients. A familial tendency to the development of aneurysms exists in 6.1% to 15.1% of IAA. IAA could be also caused by large-vessel vasculitis, particularly by giant cell arteritis and Takayasu arteritis. In published case series of Takayasu arteritis, IAA has been found in up to 45% of patients. The triad of (1) abdominal or back pain, (2) weight loss, (3) an elevated erythrocyte sedimentation rate and CRP in patients with abdominal aortic aneurysms is highly suggestive of inflammatory aneurysm. Symptoms referable to inflammatory abdominal aortic aneurysm are reported to exist in 65 to 90% of patients. This rate of presenting symptoms is significantly higher than in patients with non inflammatory abdominal aortic aneurysm, of which only 8 to 18% of patients have symptoms. Weight loss and anorexia occur in at least 20 to 41% of patients with inflammatory AAA and can be significant. One quarter of patients with inflammatory abdominal aortic aneurysm had a pulsatile abdominal mass upon examination. The aneurysm may be responsible to chronic abdominal pain and is tender to palpation. One fourth of patients have some degree of ureteral obstruction. CT scanning reliably demonstrates the characteristic thickened wall and confirms the diagnosis. Characteristic pathologic changes include infiltration of the aortic wall by lymphocytes, plasma cells, occasional multinucleated giant cells, and lymphoid follicles with germinal centers. Inflammation resolves in most cases after successful repair. Inflammatory aneurysms are easily recognized at operation by the dense, shiny, white, fibrotic material that envelops the adjacent viscera, especially the duodenum, left renal vein, and inferior vena cava. Those structures are therefore especially vulnerable to operative injury. Endovascular repair is ideal and is the procedure of choice for inflammatory aneurysms. Although inflammatory AAA appears less likely to rupture than atherosclerotic AAA, surgical intervention appears prudent once the diameter of the aneurysm exceeds 5.5 cm. Most authors agree that corticosteroids do not alter the long-term development of inflammatory aneurysms and that operative repair of the aneurysm is the treatment of choice.

10. Treatment of choice in a patient with a staghorn calculus with mild hydronephrosis:

a. ESWL
b. PCNL
c. URS
d. Open surgery

Ans. **b. PCNL**

Management options for renal stones

- Conservative management would suffice for renal stones < 5 mm in size.
- Shockwave lithotripsy is the procedure associated with the least morbidity and the lowest complication rate but is also associated with a lower success rate at treating stones as a single procedure and requires the patient to pass the stone fragments afterwards. The modality can be used for stones in the proximal ureter (particularly if <10 mm) or non-lower-pole renal stones <2 cm. The stone is located under fluoroscopic guidance, which is coupled to an extracorporeal lithotripter aimed at the stone. The stone is fragmented in a completely noninvasive manner. Complications associated with this procedure include subcapsular or perinephric renal hematoma and ureteral obstruction by stone fragments ("Steinstrausse").
- Ureteroscopy is the procedure of choice for patients with middle or distal ureteral stones. It also has a higher success rate than SWL in treating >10 mm proximal ureteral stones and renal stones. This procedure involves advancing a semi-rigid or flexible ureteroscope to the level of the stone and fragmenting it under direct visualization, often using a holmium:YAG laser. The surgeon is able to visualize the stone during fragmentation and thereby has some control over how small the fragments are. In addition, stone fragments may also be actively removed with a small nitinol stone basket. However, many patients have a ureteral stent placed after ureteroscopy, and although temporary, this remains a major source of morbidity for the patient. Specific complications of URS include ureteral injury or stricture.
- PCNL is reserved for patients with larger or more complex stone burden, and requires a percutaneous tract into the kidney. Most stones larger than 2 cm are treated with PCNL although there is a role for PCNL for smaller stones located in the lower pole of the collecting system. More powerful lithotripters (pneumatic, ultrasound) and larger instruments (stone graspers) can be used to

fragment and remove these larger stones through the percutaneous tract. Complications include injury to adjacent organs, acute and delayed renal bleeding due to pseudoaneurysm or arteriovenous fistula formation, sepsis, or renal pelvis perforation.

- Open surgical management of stones has been relegated to historic interest for the most part with less than 1% of stone surgery needing to be done open with access to modern endourologic equipment.

11. During diagnostic laparoscopy for undescended testis, the testicular vessels are found to be absent. What is the most appropriate next step?

a. Explore further
b. Nothing needs to be done
c. Inguinal exploration
d. Scrotal exploration

Ans. b. Nothing needs to be done

Cryptorchidism

Cryptorchidism or undescended testes (UDT) is a common condition occurring in 3% of full term and 30% of premature babies. Many of these testes will descend spontaneously due to the normal gonadotropin release that occurs in the first few months of life, so the true incidence is roughly 1% of boys. Untreated cryptorchidism will lead to testis damage, and there is evidence that permanent changes may occur by 3 years of age. Ideally, surgical treatment should occur prior to this age. UDT is usually an isolated finding, but it may occur as a part of a systemic condition such as Prader-Willi, Eagle-Barrett, or other such complex multisystem syndrome. Surgery is the treatment of choice; hormonal treatment has no role.

The consequences of untreated cryptorchidism include infertility and malignant degeneration. One study on fertility suggested that men with a history of unilateral cryptorchidism will have no difference in paternity rates compared to normal controls. In contrast, men with bilateral cryptorchidism have up to a 50% rate of infertility. There is data to suggest that orchidopexy in the first year of life is associated with better total sperm counts in adulthood. With regard to malignancy, untreated UDT has a fivefold increase risk of tumor development compared to the normal population. However, there is data to suggest that prepubertal orchidopexy is protective and that these boys only have a twofold greater risk.

In the case scenario given in the question, absent testicular vessels denotes that there has been intrauterine torsion and thus no further exploration is required.

12. A patient underwent thyroidectomy for hyperthyroidism. Two days later he presented with features of thyroid storm. What is the most likely cause?

a. Rough Handling of thyroid during surgery
b. Due to injury to parathyroid gland
c. Poor preoperative preparation of the patient
d. Poor antibiotic coverage

Ans. c. Poor preoperative preparation of the patient

Thyroid Storm (Thyrotoxic crisis)

- It is an emergency due to decompensated hyperthyroidism

Most common cause of thyroid storm during thyroid surgery is inadequate preparation of the patient.

Treatment

- Non-selective beta-blocker (Propranolol):
  - In thyroid storm most of the symptoms are because of adrenergic over activity due to increased tissue sensitivity to catecholamines in hyperthyroidism
  - This increased sensitivity is due to increased number of beta receptors
- Propylthiouracil:
  - It is the antithyroid drug of choice for thyrotoxicosis, because it reduces hormone synthesis as well as peripheral conversion of T4 to T3
- Corticosteroids (Hydrocortisone):
  - Inhibits both release of thyroid hormone from the gland and peripheral conversion of T4 to T3
- Iodides (Potassium iodide or Iopanoic acid):
  - Used to inhibit further hormone release from the gland
- Other measures:
  - Diltiazem, if tachycardia is not controlled by propranolol alone.
  - Rehydration, anxiolytics, external cooling & appropriate antibiotics.

13. Which of the following structures is not removed in radical neck dissection?

a. Sublingual gland
b. Submandibular gland
c. Tail of parotid gland
d. Level 2 b lymph nodes

Ans. a. Sublingual gland

Types of Cervical Lymph Node Dissections

Radical Neck Dissection

Radical neck dissection is defined as an en bloc removal of all nodal groups between the mandible and the clavicle; this removal includes the sternocleidomastoid muscle, the internal jugular vein, and the spinal accessory nerve inclusive of Zones I–V. The submandibular gland and tail of parotid gland are also removed. Since this dissection was first classified, many modifications have been proposed, especially in staging neck dissections when no palpable nodes are present.

Modified Radical Neck Dissection

A modified radical neck dissection involves sparing at least of one of these three structures—the sternocleidomastoid muscle, the internal jugular vein, or the spinal accessory nerve—while still dissecting Zones I–V. The indications for a modified radical neck dissection include definitive treatment of the neck in the presence of metastatic disease. Since the spinal accessory nerve is rarely directly involved with disease, it tends to be preserved to decrease the pain associated with shoulder dysfunction. On occasion, all three structures can be preserved if they are not directly involved with pathologic nodes.

Selective Neck Dissection

A selective neck dissection involves the preservation of one or more zones that are typically removed in a radical neck dissection. This procedure is performed when both the treatment of the primary lesion is surgical and the risk of occult metastasis to the cervical lymph nodes is greater than 20%.

Supraomohyoid neck dissection—Involves Zones I–III and is usually performed in conjunction with oral cavity tumors and N0 neck disease. Its most common role is in the dissection of the contralateral neck at high risk for cervical metastasis in order to avoid postoperative radiation therapy.

Lateral compartment neck dissection—Zones II–IV; it is used in conjunction with the surgical resection of tumors of the larynx, hypopharynx, and pharynx.

Posterolateral neck dissection—Include Zones II–V and include nodes in the retroauricular and suboccipital regions. These dissections are often performed when cutaneous malignant tumors metastasize to the neck.

Anterior compartment neck dissection—Includes Zone VI and is used for tumors found in the larynx, hypopharynx, subglottis, cervical esophagus, and thyroid. It includes the removal of the thyroid lobe and necessitates both the identification and the preservation of the parathyroid glands, with reimplantation as needed.

Extended Radical Neck Dissection

Extended neck dissections involve the additional removal of muscle, nerves, vessels, and lymph node groups as dictated by the primary disease and the presence of metastasis.

14. A chronic alcoholic presents to the ED with epigastric pain and recurrent vomiting. On examination, he has guarding in epigastrium. Chest radiograph is normal. What is the next best step?

a. UGI endoscopy
b. Serum lipase
c. CECT
d. Alcohol breath test

Ans. **b. Serum lipase**

Clinical Approach to Suspected Acute Pancreatitis

Patients with acute pancreatitis usually complain of sudden onset unrelenting epigastric pain that is sharp in nature. This pain often radiates to the back. Nausea and vomiting are common as is anorexia. Patients may present with signs of volume depletion in the setting of decreased oral intake as well as potential third-space losses. Signs of systemic inflammation are common at the time of presentation including fever, tachycardia, and leukocytosis. Rarely, physical examination findings may include evidence of hemorrhagic pancreatitis such as flank (Gray-Turner sign) or periumbilical (Cullen sign) ecchymosis.

The presence of epigastric pain with an elevation in amylase/lipase ≥ 3 times normal is highly accurate for the diagnosis of acute pancreatitis. Additional considerations should include acute cholecystitis or ascending cholangitis (both of which may be concurrent with an attack of biliary pancreatitis). Less common considerations include a penetrating duodenal ulcer, bowel ischemia, renal colic, or diabetic ketoacidosis. Further potentially life-threatening conditions include a perforated viscus, bowel obstruction or myocardial infarction. Serum amylase may also be elevated in salivary disorders, ectopic pregnancy, or macroamylasemia.

The diagnosis of acute pancreatitis requires at least two of the following: (1) typical epigastric abdominal pain, (2) amylase/lipase evaluation ≥ 3 times upper limit of normal, and/or (3) confirmatory findings on cross-sectional imaging. Findings on abdominal ultrasound in conjunction with liver function tests have very high sensitivity for the detection of gallstone-related illness. Specifically, an elevated ALT level > 2 to 3 times normal has been found to have a 95% positive predictive value for gallstone-related illness.

15. Most common functional tumor of endocrine pancreas:

a. VIPoma
b. Gastrinoma
c. Glucagonoma
d. Somatostatinoma

Ans. **b. Gastrinoma**

Insulinoma is the most common functional tumor but since it is not given in the options, gastrinoma is the best answer.

Islet Cell Tumors (Pancreatic Neuroendocrine Tumors)

Islet cell tumors may be nonfunctional, hypofunctional, or hyperfunctional with respect to their progenitor specific hormone-secreting cells (beta, alpha, and delta). If nonfunctional, they may only present with symptoms of a mass lesion, sometimes only discovered incidentally. Functional islet cell tumors secrete a variety of hormones; in descending order of frequency, they are the following: gastrin, insulin, serotonin, and vasoactive intestinal peptide (VIP). The cell types and their respective hormones are summarized below:

Beta cell tumors (insulinoma) are clinically significant when they produce enough insulin to induce hypoglycemia (discussed below). Laboratory studies include blood glucose, C-peptide, insulin, and the insulin to glucose ratio.

Alpha cell tumors (glucagonoma) are associated with elevated serum levels of glucagon. These tumors can be associated with a characteristic migratory erythema, as well as glucose intolerance, weight loss, deep vein thrombosis, and depression.

Delta cell tumors (somatostatinoma) are typically associated with diabetes-related symptoms, diarrhea, steatorrhea, cholelithiasis, and weight loss. These tumors are most often located in the duodenum or jejunum, rather than in the pancreas.

Tumors of the pancreatic islets that secrete gastrin (gastrinoma) are found in both pancreas and duodenum with a higher incidence in the pancreas (60% to 85% depending on source reviewed) with 90% of them occurring in the "gastrinoma triangle," a triangle with its base parallel to the cystic duct and its apex pointing toward the tail. Gastrin elevations are associated with increased gastric acid secretion, diarrhea, and malabsorption (Zollinger–Ellison syndrome). Patients with peptic ulcer disease without *Helicobacter pylori* infection or a history of nonsteroidal anti-inflammatory drug use may have Zollinger–Ellison syndrome and should be evaluated for a gastrinoma.

Lastly, VIP-secreting tumors are known as VIPomas. VIPomas induce a syndrome of watery diarrhea, hypokalemia, hypochlorhydria, and acidosis.

16. True/False about Prostate cancer:

a. It commonly arises from central zone
b. Histological grading by Gleason's score
c. Most common type of prostate cancer is squamous cell type
d. It is hormone dependent

Ans. a-F, b-T, c-F, d-T

- Prostatic carcinoma arises from posterior lobe and peripheral zone.
- BPH arises from medial lobe and transitional zone.
- Classification of histological pattern based on the degree of glandular de-differentiation and its relation to stroma has been devised by Gleason. Gleason score 8-10; High grade tumor and poor prognosis. Gleason score 2–10 helps to predict the like hood of spared and prognosis.

Prostatic Cancer

- Prostatic cancer is the most common malignant tumor in men over 65 years of age.
- Symptoms of bladder outlet obstruction and back pains (due to bony metastasis in the pelvis and lumber vertebra) indicate toward prostate cancer.
- Most common metastatic sites of prostate carcinoma are lymph nodes are bones.
- Lymphatic metastasis occurs most commonly to → obturator lymph nodes.
- Most common bony metastasis occurs in: Lumber spine (most common) > Proximal femur > Pelvis > Thoracic spine > ribs
- Most effective screening protocol: Combination of digital rectal examination and serum PSA monitoring.
- Tumors marker in Prostate carcinoma:
  - Serum acid phosphate is a tumor marker of prostate cancer.
  - But now serum acid phosphate assay has been suppressed by PSA assay (Prostate specific antigen).

Treatment

- *Radical prostatectomy*: Removal of prostate and seminal vesicle up to distal sphincter mechanism.
- High chances of urinary incontinence and retrograde ejaculation is seen after surgery
- This surgery is possible only in T1 and T2 cases.
- T3 and T4 cases treatment is only palliative
- Radical radiotherapy is equally beneficial in T1 and T2 cases.

17. On 5th postoperative day of CABG, patient develops tachypnea and hypertension. What is the most probable cause?

a. Sepsis
b. Acute kidney failure
c. Acute respiratory failure
d. Acute cardiac failure

Ans. **d. Acute cardiac failure**

Complications after CABG

A number of complications are associated with coronary artery bypass grafting (CABG), both in the short term and in the long term; they are associated with anesthesia, cardiopulmonary bypass, sternotomy, and the operation itself. These complications may include the following:

- Myocardial dysfunction
- Cerebrovascular complications
- Acute renal failure
- Cardiac tamponade
- Respiratory tract infections
- Aortic dissection

In the initial postoperative period, there is a decline in myocardial function secondary to myocardial edema and ischemia-reperfusion injury. Additional factors (e.g., incomplete revascularization and postoperative graft failure) may exacerbate the dysfunction. Patients may exhibit a low-output syndrome, with 4–9% requiring the use of inotropes or intra-aortic balloon pulsation. Additionally, segmental transmural myocardial infarction occurs in 1–5% of patients, and postoperative arrhythmias occur in approximately 30% of patients after CABG.

Adverse neurologic outcomes are a major concern in cardiac surgery, with 3.1% for major (type I) events (e.g., major neurologic deficits and coma) occurring in 3.1% of cases, and 3% for less-debilitating (type II) events (deterioration of intellectual function or memory). Both types of events result in a significant increase in mortality: 21% for type I events and 10% for type II. Despite the increased mortality associated with type II events, the majority of survivors return to normal activity in the following 3–12 months.

Postoperative renal failure is a significant cause of mortality after CABG. There is a 4% incidence of renal failure; 20% of these patients require dialysis, and the mortality is 50%.

18. Identify the name of the disease shown here in the breast?

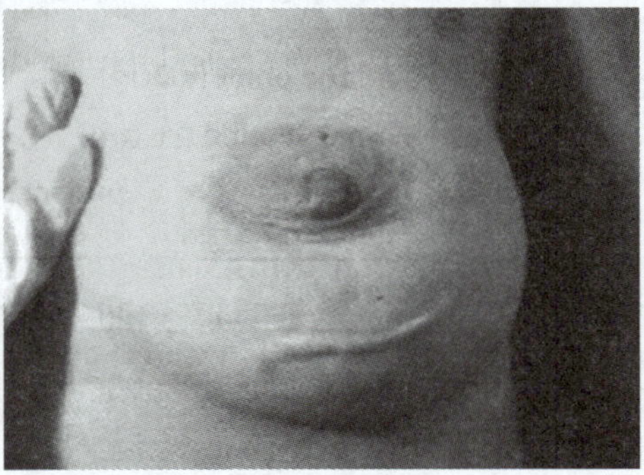

a. Pagets disease
b. Mondor's disease
c. Red manhood
d. Tietze syndrome

Ans. b. Mondor's disease

Mondor's Disease

Thrombophlebitis of the superficial thoracoepigastric vein, or Mondor's disease, results in a cordlike mass in the breast, sometimes associated with skin changes such as dimpling. Although no identifiable cause is found in most cases, localized trauma or an inflammatory process has been associated with Mondor's disease. Breast pain is the usual presenting complaint, with examination findings of a characteristic cordlike mass in the superficial subcutaneous tissue of the breast, most commonly in the lower quadrants. Mondor's disease, which can be mistaken for an inflammatory cancer, is benign and self-limited. US can establish the diagnosis of superficial thrombophlebitis. Past treatment was nonsteroidal anti-inflammatory medication. Consider thrombophilic evaluation and treatment with low-molecular-weight heparins after hematology consultation.

Obstetrics and Gynecology

1. A 30 years old G3P2 patient visits an antenatal clinic at 20 weeks. She reveals during history that her first baby weighed 4.6 kg, second baby weighed 4.8 kg and both were delivered by C-section. The gynecologist suspects gestational diabetes and orders a GTT. The blood sugar level after 50 gm of oral glucose are 206 mg% and the patient is thus confirmed as a case of gestational diabetes. All of the following are known complications of this condition *except*?

a. Susceptibility for infection
b. Fetal hyperglycemia
c. Congenital malformation in fetus
d. Neonatal hypoglycemia

Ans. **b. Fetal hyperglycemia**

Diabetes Mellitus During Pregnancy

Maternal Complications

- Recurrent abortions in uncontrolled diabetes
- Preterm labor because of infection, Polyhydramnios
- Recurrent UTIs
- Increased incidence of pre-eclampsia
- Polyhydramnios
- Prolongation of labor due to big baby
- Shoulder dystocia
- Perineal injuries, postpartum hemorrhage
- *Puerperium*: Puerperal sepsis, lactation failure

Fetal Complications

- Fetal macrosomia (30–40%) due to maternal hyperglycemia and elevation of maternal free fatty acids
- Congenital malformations (6–10%) are seen in uncontrolled overt diabetes mellitus
- *CNS and skeletal*: NTD, anencephaly, microcephaly, sacral agenesis
- *Cardiac*: VSD, ASD, coarctation of aorta, transposition of great vessels
- *Renal*: Renal agenesis, hydronephrosis, ureteral duplication
- *GIT*: Duodenal atresia, anorectal atresia
- *Others*: Single umbilical artery
- Most common congenital malformation is congenital heart disease, most common being VSD
- Most specific congenital heart disease associated with maternal diabetes is TGA
- Most specific congenital malformation is sacral agenesis (Caudal regression syndrome)

Neonatal Complications

- Hypoglycemia
- Respiratory distress syndrome
- Hyperbilirubinemia
- Polycythemia
- Hypocalcemia
- Hypomagnesemia
- Cardiomyopathy

Maternal hyperglycemia and diabetes associated macrosomia are associated with increased risk of intrauterine fetal death and other adverse outcomes. Induction of labor may be considered at 38–39 weeks, although there is no good-quality evidence to support such an approach. As diabetic pregnancies are associated with a delay in lung maturity, we must choose a time which balances the risk of sudden intrauterine fetal death and the risk of neonatal respiratory distress due to lung immaturity. If the option 39 weeks is given, this should be chosen.

In case of fetal macrosomia (estimated fetal weight >4 kg) consideration should be given for a primary cesarean section at 39 weeks to avoid shoulder dystocia. In pregnant women with GDM with poor blood sugar control, those with risk factors like hypertensive disorder of pregnancy, previous stillbirth and other complications should be delivered earlier. The timing of delivery should be individualized.

Gestational diabetes which is controlled on diet and exercise alone may be prolonged till 40 weeks.

2. A pregnant lady is suffering from SLE. Which of the following autoantibodies would be responsible if her child has congenital heart block?

a. Anti-Sm
b. Anti-dsDNA
c. Antiphospholipid antibody
d. Anti-Rho

Ans. d. Anti-Rho

Autoantibodies in Systemic Lupus Erythematosus (SLE)

Antibody	Prevalence, %	Antigen Recognized	Clinical Utility
Antinuclear antibodies	98	Multiple nuclear	Best screening test; repeated negative tests by immunofluorescence make SLE unlikely
Anti-dsDNA	70	DNA (double-stranded)	High titers are SLE-specific and in some patients correlate with disease activity, nephritis, vasculitis. Crithidia immunofluorescence is more specific for SLE than ELISA methods.

Contd...

Contd...

Antibody	Prevalence, %	Antigen Recognized	Clinical Utility
Anti-Sm	25	Protein complexed to 6 species of nuclear U1 RNA	Specific for SLE; no definite clinical correlations; most patients also have anti-RNP; more common in blacks and Asians than whites
Anti-RNP	40	Protein complexed to U1 RNA	Not specific for SLE; high titers associated with syndromes that have overlap features of several rheumatic syndromes including SLE; more common in blacks than whites; correlates with high IFN-induced gene signature
Anti-Ro (SS-A)	30	Protein complexed to hY RNA, primarily 60 kDa and 52 kDa	Not specific for SLE; associated with sicca syndrome, predisposes to subacute cutaneous lupus, and to neonatal lupus with congenital heart block; associated with decreased risk for nephritis
Anti-La (SS-B)	10	47-kDa protein complexed to hY RNA	Usually associated with anti-Ro; associated with decreased risk for nephritis
Antihistone	70	Histones associated with DNA (in nucleosome, chromatin)	More frequent in drug-induced lupus than in SLE
Antiphospholipid	50	Phospholipids, β_2 glycoprotein 1 (β_2G1) cofactor, prothrombin	Three tests available—ELISAs for cardiolipin and β_2G1, sensitive prothrombin time (DRVVT) for lupus anticoagulant; predisposes to clotting, fetal loss, thrombocytopenia
Antierythrocyte	60	Erythrocyte membrane	Measured as direct Coombs test; a small proportion develops overt hemolysis
Antiplatelet	30	Surface and altered cytoplasmic antigens on platelets	Associated with thrombocytopenia, but sensitivity and specificity are not good; this is not a useful clinical test

Contd...

Contd...

Antibody	Prevalence, %	Antigen Recognized	Clinical Utility
Antineuronal (includes antiglutamate receptor 2)	60	Neuronal and lymphocyte surface antigens	In some series, a positive test in CSF correlates with active CNS lupus
Antiribosomal P	20	Protein in ribosomes	In some series, a positive test in serum correlates with depression or psychosis due to CNS lupus

3. Arrange the following antenatal investigations in sequential order:

a. NTNB scan
b. Anomaly scan
c. Growth scan
d. Triple marker test

Ans. a. NTNB scan, **d.** Triple marker test, **b.** Anomaly scan, **c.** Growth scan

Tests Used for Detection of Congenital Anomalies

Test	Performed at	Detection rate	False positive	Description
Triple test	15–20 weeks	70%	5%	Maternal serum AFP (Low) + Estriol (Low) + hCG (High)
Quad screen	15–20 weeks	81%	5%	Triple test + Inhibin-alpha (High)
First trimester Combined test	10–13 weeks	85%	5%	Ultrasound to measure: Nuchal translucency (Increased) Ductus venosus flow (reversed) Nasal bone (hypoplasia) + hCG + PAPP-A (Pregnancy associated plasma protein A)

Contd...

Contd...

Test	Performed at	Detection rate	False positive	Description
Integrated test	10–13 weeks and 15–20 weeks	95%	5%	Measurements from both the 1st trimester combined test & 2nd trimester Quad test to yield a more accurate screening result.
Level II scan/ anomaly scan	18–22 weeks			Detailed evaluation of all organs of the fetus for detection of anomalies

Growth scan is performed in the 3rd trimester for assessing the growth parameters of the fetus.

4. Which of the following drugs has neuroprotective action on the fetus when used in preterm birth?

a. $MgSO_4$ b. Oxytocin
c. Nicardipine d. Salbutamol

Ans. **a. $MgSO_4$**

Magnesium Sulfate for Fetal/Neonatal Neuroprotection

Several recent large trials have shown a reduced risk of cerebral palsy in fetuses exposed to magnesium sulfate in utero. The largest trial from the United States demonstrated a significant reduction in moderate to severe cerebral palsy in children at or beyond 2 years of age who received magnesium sulfate immediately before delivery. The optimal candidates for magnesium for this indication are not well defined, but it is reasonable to offer magnesium sulfate to any woman between 23 0/7 and 32 0/7 weeks of gestation immediately before delivery to reduce the risk of adverse neurologic outcomes in the neonate.

Protocol for use of magnesium sulfate for fetal neuroprotection:

Criteria for Admission

- Preterm birth anticipated within 2–24 hours.
- Gestational age of 24–31 6/7 weeks has been confirmed.
- Any specific contraindications to magnesium sulfate therapy have been ruled out.

Protocol

- Begin intravenous infusion of magnesium sulfate loading dose, 6 g over 20–30 minutes, followed by a maintenance infusion of 2 g per hour.

- If delivery has not occurred after 12 hours and is no longer considered imminent, the infusion may be discontinued.
- If > 6 hours has passed since discontinuation of magnesium sulfate and delivery is again believed to be imminent, another loading dose may be given followed by maintenance infusion.

5. What is the best treatment for impending eclampsia at 35 weeks period of gestation?

a. Steroids
b. Emergency cesarean section
c. Induce labor
d. Magnesium sulfate

Ans. c. Induce labor

Preeclampsia

Early recognition is the key to treatment. The objectives are to prolong pregnancy if possible to allow fetal lung maturity while preventing progression to severe disease and eclampsia. The critical factors are the gestational age of the fetus, fetal pulmonary maturity, and the severity of maternal disease. Preeclampsia-eclampsia at term is managed by delivery. Prior to term, severe preeclampsia-eclampsia requires delivery with very few exceptions. Epigastric pain, seizures, severe range blood pressures, thrombocytopenia, and visual disturbances are strong indications for delivery of the fetus. Marked proteinuria alone can be managed more conservatively.

Hospitalization is required for women with preeclampsia with severe features. Regular assessments of blood pressure, urine protein, and fetal heart tones and activity are required. A CBC with platelet count, electrolyte panel, and liver enzymes should be checked regularly, with frequency dependent on severity. A 24-hour urine collection for total protein and creatinine clearance should be obtained on admission and repeated as indicated. Magnesium sulfate is not used until the diagnosis of severe preeclampsia is made and delivery planned.

Fetal evaluation should be obtained as part of the workup. This may be done by fetal heart rate testing with nonstress testing or by biophysical profile. If the fetus is less than 34 weeks' gestation, corticosteroids (betamethasone 12 mg intramuscularly every 24 h for two doses, or dexamethasone 6 mg intramuscularly every 12 h for four doses) can be administered to the mother. However, when a woman is clearly suffering from unstable severe preeclampsia, delivery should not be delayed for fetal lung maturation or administration of corticosteroids.

The method of delivery is determined by the maternal and fetal status. A vaginal delivery is preferred because it has less blood loss than a cesarean section and requires less coagulation factors. Cesarean section is reserved for the usual fetal indications. For mild preeclampsia, delivery should take place at term.

Eclampsia

Emergency care: If the patient is convulsing, she is turned on her side to prevent aspiration and to improve blood flow to the placenta. The seizure may be stopped by giving an intravenous bolus of either magnesium sulfate, 4–6 g, or lorazepam, 2–4 mg over 4 minutes or until the seizure stops. Magnesium sulfate is the preferred agent, and alternatives should be used only if magnesium sulfate is unavailable. A continuous intravenous infusion of magnesium sulfate is then started at a rate of 2–3 g/h unless the patient is known to have significantly reduced kidney function. Magnesium blood levels are then checked every 4–6 hours and the infusion rate adjusted to maintain a therapeutic blood level (4–7 mEq/L). Urinary output is checked hourly and the patient assessed for signs of possible magnesium toxicity such as loss of deep tendon reflexes or decrease in respiratory rate and depth, which can be reversed with calcium gluconate, 1 g intravenously over 2 minutes.

General care: In patients who have preeclampsia with severe features, magnesium sulfate should be given intravenously, 4- to 6-g load over 15–20 minutes followed by 2–3 g/h maintenance, for seizure prophylaxis. The occurrence of eclampsia necessitates delivery once the patient is stabilized. Continuous fetal monitoring must be performed and maternal blood typed and cross-matched quickly. If hypertension is present with systolic values of 160 mm Hg or higher or diastolic values 110 mm Hg or higher, antihypertensive medications should be administered to reduce the blood pressure to 140–150/90–100 mm Hg. Hydralazine given in 5- to 10-mg increments intravenously every 20 minutes is frequently used to lower blood pressure. Labetalol, 10–20 mg intravenously, every 20 minutes as needed, can also be used.

Delivery: Delivery is mandated once eclampsia has occurred. Vaginal delivery is preferred. Cesarean section is used for the usual obstetric indications.

Postpartum: Magnesium sulfate infusion (2–3 g/h) should be continued for 24 hours postpartum.

6. Multiple correct type. Uterotonic drugs amongst the following are:

a. Oxytocin
b. Misoprostol
c. PGF_{2a}
d. Dinoprostone
e. None

Ans. **a-T, b-T, c-T, d-F**

Postpartum Hemorrhage

Immediate steps

1. Cell for help including seniors. Alert consultant obstetrician, hematologist, anesthetist and senior midwives or nurses.
2. Resuscitation. Start I.V. line with two 14 G cannulae
3. Send blood for hemogram, platelet count, bleeding and coagulation profile, urea, electrolytes, liver function tests
4. Arrange at least 2 units each of PRBC, fresh frozen plasma, platelets, cryoprecipitates
5. Warm the blood bank that more blood and blood products may be required.
6. Fast infusion of normal saline Hartman's solution or Ringer lactate or hemaccel up to 2 L till blood reaches
7. Catheterize with Foley's catheter
8. Keep patient warm
9. Start oxygen
10. Consider central line for major PPH
11. ECG and Oximeter

↓

Find out cause of PPH by abdominal palpation

↓

Uterus atonic (Atonic PPH)

1. Uterine massage
2. Inj. Methergin 0.2 mg I.V. every 2-4 hours
3. Oxytocin infusion 40 units in 500 mL of normal saline, at the rate of 40–60 drops per minute.
4. Empty the bladder
5. Ensure complete uterine evacuation
6. Blood transfusion
7. Weigh all swabs and estimate blood loss

↓

Uterus still atonic

1. Give 250 μg of carboprost I.M. every 15 minutes for 8 doses
2. Give 500 μg of carboprost intramyometrially
3. Give 800 μg misoprostol rectally

↓

Uterine tamponade

1. Bimanual uterine compression or
2. Intrauterine packing with 5 metres x 8 cm gauze under anesthesia or
3. Insertion of a Sengstaken-Blakemore Esophageal catheter (SBEC) or Bakri balloon or condom catheter
4. Consider military antishock treatment or garment (MAST)
5. Continue blood transfusion and uterotonics

↓

Uterus still atonic

↓

Consider surgery

1. Brace sutures (B-Lynch) Hayman sutures or Cho's sutures
2. Bilateral uterine and utero ovarian arteries ligation
3. Bilateral anterior division or internal iliac artery ligation
4. Uterine artery embolization

↓

Hysterectomy as a last resort → Shift the patient to intensive care unit or high dependency unit

Uterus hard and well contracted (Traumatic PPH)

↓

Resuscitation with fluids and blood as above Catheterization of bladder

↓

- Exploration (Cervico-vaginal inspection) → Hemostatic sutures on the tear sites (stitching of perineal, vaginal and cervical tears)
- Suspicion of uterine rupture → Emergency laparotomy → Hysterectomy (sub-total or total)

7. A young lady presents to the gynecology OPD with complaints of primary infertility, excessive weight gain and hirsutism. Laparoscopy shows the following finding. What is the most likely diagnosis?

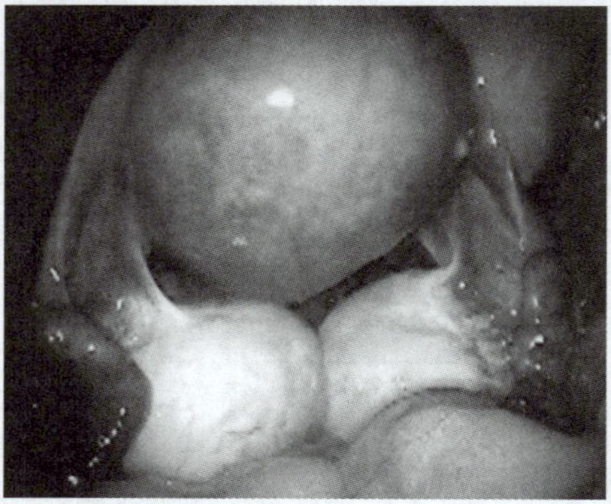

a. Turner's syndrome
b. Pituitary adenoma
c. PCOS
d. Bilateral dysgerminoma

Ans. c. PCOS

Laparoscopic image shows bilaterally enlarged ovaries.

Polycystic ovary syndrome:

PCOS is a common functional disorder of the ovaries of unknown etiology. It accounts for at least 50% of all cases of hirsutism associated with elevated serum testosterone levels. It is familial and transmitted as a complex polygenic disorder whose phenotypic expression may involve both protective and susceptible genomic variants.

A diagnosis of PCOS must meet three criteria: (1) androgen excess with clinical hyperandrogenism or elevated serum free or total testosterone; (2) ovarian dysfunction with oligoanovulation or polycystic ovary morphology; and (3) absence of other causes of testosterone excess or anovulation such as pregnancy, thyroid dysfunction, 21-hydroxylase deficiency, neoplastic testosterone secretion, Cushing syndrome, or hyperprolactinemia.

Affected women usually have signs of hyperandrogenism, including hirsutism, acne, or male-pattern thinning of scalp hair; this persists after natural menopause. Most women also have elevated serum testosterone or free testosterone levels. About 70% of affected women have polycystic ovaries on pelvic ultrasound and 50% have oligomenorrhea or amenorrhea with anovulation. Of note, about 30% of women with PCOS do not have cystic ovaries and 25–30% of normal menstruating women have cystic ovaries.

Obesity and high serum insulin levels (due to insulin resistance) contribute to the syndrome in 70% of women. The serum LH:FSH ratio is often greater than 2.0. Both adrenal and ovarian androgen hypersecretion are commonly present. Diabetes mellitus is present in about 13% of cases. Untreated women with amenorrhea have a slightly increased risk of endometrial carcinoma. Hypertension and hyperlipidemia are often present, increasing the risk of cardiovascular disease.

USG features: In patients >8 years post menarche, and using a high-frequency endovaginal probe:

- Follicle number per ovary (FNPO) ≥ 20, and/or
- Ovarian volume ≥10 mL, ensuring no corpora lutea, cysts or dominant follicles are present.

If using transabdominal scanning, or older technology where ovarian morphology is not well visualized, consider using the ovarian volume threshold of ≥10 mL on either ovary.

The diagnostic criteria are adjusted in adolescent females (defined as within 8 years of menarche, or age <20 years), in whom ultrasound should not be used for the diagnosis of PCOS due to the high incidence of multi-follicular ovaries in this life stage. This supersedes the initial Rotterdam criteria of ≥12 follicles and interim recommendations of 24 or 25 follicles per ovary. The presence of a single multifollicular ovary is sufficient to provide the sonographic criterion for PCOS.

Other morphological features have been described, but do not contribute to formal diagnostic criteria:

- Hyperechoic central stroma
- Peripheral location of follicles (string of pearls sign)
- Follicles of similar size measuring 2–9 mm

8. A 35 years old lady presents with post-coital bleed. On examination, there is presence of cervical hypertrophy and anterior erosion with a healthy vagina. What will be next step in management?

a. PAP smear
b. Conization
c. Four quadrant biopsy
d. Hysterectomy

Ans. c. Four quadrant biopsy

- Post-coital bleeding is highly suggestive of carcinoma of cervix in the absence of genital tract infection. Colposcopy guided biopsy is the best method for diagnosis. However, in the absence of colposcopy facility, a four-quadrant biopsy can be done for confirming the diagnosis.
- Pap smear is a screening test and we cannot comment on invasion. HSIL (high-grade squamous intraepithelial lesion), which is diagnosed

on pap smear cytology should be followed by a colposcopy, a cervical biopsy and endocervical assessment.

- Further management is based on histopathology of the cervical biopsy taken. If it is CIN-3, we must perform a diagnostic excisional procedure such as LEEP to diagnose any invasion.
- Conization is a diagnostic excisional procedure which at times also represents adequate treatment for CIN-3 (in young women). However, it must be preceded by colposcopy and cervical biopsy.

9. A patient presents with heavy menstrual bleeding. Hysteroscopy was done, which revealed the following finding. What is the most likely diagnosis?

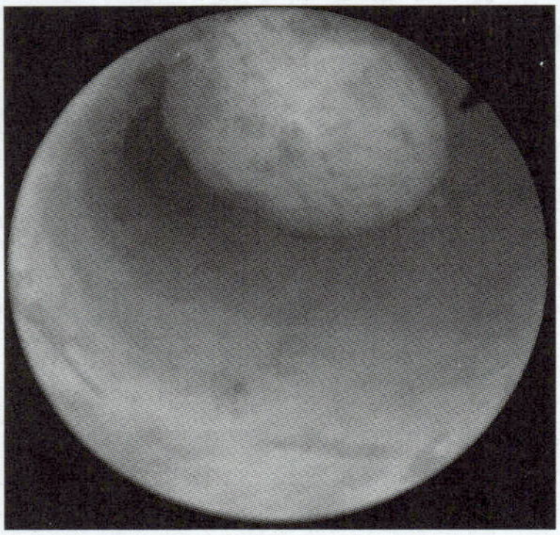

a. Asherman syndrome b. Cervical carcinoma
c. Endometrial carcinoma d. Submucosal fibroid

Ans. d. Submucosal fibroid

Uterine Fibroid

- Uterine leiomyoma is the most common benign neoplasm of the female genital tract
- It is a discrete, round, firm, often multiple uterine tumor composed of smooth muscle and connective tissue
- The most convenient classification is by anatomic location:
  - Intramural
  - Submucous
  - Subserous
  - Intraligamentous
  - Parasitic (i.e., deriving its blood supply from an organ to which it becomes attached)
  - Cervical
- Symptoms and Signs
  - Frequently asymptomatic in nonpregnant women

- Abnormal uterine bleeding and pelvic pain or pressure most common symptoms
- Occasionally, degeneration occurs, causing intense pain
- The risk of miscarriage is increased if the myoma significantly distorts the uterine cavity and interferes with implantation
- Fibroids rarely cause infertility by leading to bilateral tubal blockage; they more commonly cause miscarriage and pregnancy complications, such as preterm labor, preterm delivery, and malpresentation

- Investigations
  - *Ultrasonography*: Confirms presence of uterine myomas; can be used sequentially to monitor growth
  - *MRI*: Can delineate intramural and submucous myomas accurately; necessary prior to uterine artery embolization to assess blood flow to the fibroids
  - *Diagnostic procedures*: Hysterography or hysteroscopy can also confirm cervical or submucous myomas.

Treatment

Emergency Measures

- Emergency surgery may be required for acute torsion of a pedunculated myoma
- If the patient is markedly anemic as a result of long, heavy menstrual periods, preoperative treatment with following medications will slow or stop bleeding
- DMPA—150 mg intramuscularly every 3 months
- Depot leuprolide—3.75 mg intramuscularly monthly
- Nafarelin—0.2–0.4 mg intranasally twice daily
- Levonorgestrel—containing IUDs have also been used to decrease the bleeding associated with fibroids; however, IUD placement can be more technically challenging in patients with fibroids
- The only emergency indication for myomectomy during pregnancy is torsion of a pedunculated fibroid.

Specific Measures

- Women who have small asymptomatic myomas can be managed expectantly and evaluated annually
- In patients wishing to defer surgical management, nonhormonal therapies (such as NSAIDs and tranexamic acid) have been shown to decrease menstrual blood loss
- Hormonal therapies such as GnRH agonists and selective progesterone receptor modulators (SPRMs), such as low-dose mifepristone (5–10 mg/day) have been shown to reduce myoma volume, uterine size, and menstrual blood loss.

Surgical Measures

- Surgical intervention is based on the patient's symptoms and desire for future fertility.
- Uterine size alone is not an indication for surgery
- Cervical myomas larger than 3–4 cm in diameter or pedunculated myomas that protrude through the cervix can cause bleeding, infection, degeneration, pain, or urinary retention and often require removal
- Submucous myomas can be removed by hysteroscopic resection
- Myomectomy is the treatment of choice for women who wish to preserve fertility
- Uterine artery embolization: Minimally invasive treatment for uterine fibroids; Goal is to block the blood vessels supplying the fibroids, causing them to shrink.

10. What is the best treatment option for metropathia hemorrhagica?

a. Cyclical progesterone b. Hysterectomy
c. Uterine artery embolization d. Dilatation and curettage

Ans. **a. Cyclical progesterone**

Metropathia hemorrhagica

- It is a special form of dysfunctional uterine bleeding
- It is characterized by thickening of the endometrium and cystic follicles in one or both ovaries
- It is most commonly seen in women over 40 years of age, however it may also develop in young girls.

Clinical findings:

- Most common complaint is continuous vaginal bleeding which may last for weeks
- Bleeding is always painless since it is anovulatory.

It is subdivided into 3 types based upon the menstrual history:

- Type 1: Occurs in 50% cases; continuous vaginal bleeding is preceded by amenorrhea of about 8 to 10 weeks
- Type 2: Bleeding follows normal pattern and occurs at the normal expected time
- Type 3: Bleeding may be preceded by menorrhagia

Differential diagnosis are—ectopic gestation and miscarriage:

Treatment: Cyclical progesterone therapy.

11. Mark the following statements as true or false with respect to the indications of hormone replacement therapy after menopause:

a. It is effective for vasomotor symptoms during perimenopausal period
b. It should be given for young women with premature menopause
c. It is useful for primary prevention of heart disease

d. Cyclical HRT is preferred over continuous HRT in perimenopausal women
e. None

Ans. a-T, b-T, c-F, d-T

Hormone Replacement Therapy

- The main indication of HRT is vasomotor and other symptoms in the perimenopausal period.
- It should be used at the smallest effective dose and for the shortest duration.
- Young women with premature menopause clearly deserve HRT.
- Hysterectomized women should receive estrogen alone, while those with intact uterus should be given estrogen + progestin.
- Perimenopausal women should be given cyclic HRT rather than continuous HRT.
- HRT is not the best option to prevent osteoporosis and fractures.
- HRT affords no protection against cardiovascular diseases conventional dose combined HRT. It may evenincrease the risk of venous thromboembolism, MI and stroke.
- HRT does not protect against cognitive decline; may increase the risk of dementia.
- Combined HRT increases the risk of breast cancer, gallstones and migraine.
- Transdermal HRT may have certain advantages over oral HRT.
- The need for HRT should be assessed in individual women, and not prescribed routinely.
- *Subject*: OBG
- *Topic*: Menopause and HRT

12. Assertion: Hot flushes are common after menopause
Reason: Estrogen withdrawal happens in menopause

a. Both Assertion and Reasoning are independently true/correct and Reason is the correct explanation of the Assertion
b. Both Assertion and Reasoning are independently true/correct and Reason is not the correct explanation of the Assertion
c. Assertion is independently a true/correct statement but the Reason is independently an incorrect/false statement
d. Assertion is independently a false/incorrect statement but the Reason is independently a true/correct statement
e. Both Assertion and Reason are independently a false/incorrect statement

Ans. a. Both Assertion and Reasoning are independently true/correct and Reason is the correct explanation of the Assertion

Menopause

The term "menopause" denotes the final cessation of menstruation, either as a normal part of aging or as the result of surgical removal of both ovaries. In a broader sense, as the term is commonly used, it denotes a 1- to 3-year period during which a woman adjusts to a diminishing and then absent menstrual flow and the physiologic changes that may be associated with lowered estrogen levels—hot flushes, night sweats, and vaginal dryness.

The average age at menopause is 51 years. Premature menopause is defined as ovarian failure and menstrual cessation before age 40; this often has a genetic or autoimmune basis. Surgical menopause due to bilateral oophorectomy is common and can cause more severe symptoms owing to the sudden rapid drop in sex hormone levels.

Clinical findings:

1. *Cessation of menstruation*: Menstrual cycles generally become irregular as menopause approaches. Anovular cycles occur more often, with irregular cycle length and occasional menorrhagia. Menstrual flow usually diminishes in amount owing to decreased estrogen secretion, resulting in less abundant endometrial growth. Finally, cycles become longer, with missed periods or episodes of spotting only. When no bleeding has occurred for 1 year, the menopausal transition can be said to have occurred.
2. *Hot flushes*: Hot flushes (feelings of intense heat over the trunk and face, with flushing of the skin and sweating) occur in over 80% of women as a result of the decrease in ovarian hormones. Hot flushes can begin before the cessation of menses. Menopausal vasomotor symptoms last longer than previously thought, and there are ethnic differences in the duration of symptoms. Vasomotor symptoms were found to last more than 7 years in more than 50% of the women.
3. *Vaginal atrophy*: With decreased estrogen secretion, thinning of the vaginal mucosa and decreased vaginal lubrication occur and may lead to dyspareunia. The introitus decreases in diameter. Pelvic examination reveals pale, smooth vaginal mucosa and a small cervix and uterus.
4. *Osteoporosis*: Osteoporosis may occur as a late sequela of menopause

13. Which of the following types of trophoblast cells invade the spiral arterioles?

a. Villous
b. Endovascular
c. Interstitial
d. None of the above

Ans. b. Endovascular

Trophoblast Development

Human placental formation begins with the trophectoderm, which gives rise to a trophoblast cell layer encircling the blastocyst. From then until term, trophoblasts play a critical part at the fetal–maternal interface. Trophoblasts exhibit the most variable structure, function, and developmental pattern of all placental components. Their invasiveness promotes implantation, their nutritional role for the conceptus is reflected in their name, and their endocrine organ function is essential to maternal physiological adaptations and to pregnancy maintenance.

By the eighth day postfertilization, after initial implantation, trophoblasts have differentiated into an outer multinucleated syncytium—primitive *syncytiotrophoblast*, and an inner layer of primitive mononuclear cells—*cytotrophoblasts*. The latter are germinal cells for the syncytium. As cytotrophoblasts proliferate, their cell walls disappear, and the cells fuse to add to the expanding outer layer of syncytiotrophoblast. Each cytotrophoblast has a well-demarcated cell border, a single nucleus, and ability to undergo DNA synthesis and mitosis. These are lacking in the syncytiotrophoblast, which provides transport functions of the placenta. It is so named because instead of individual cells, it has an amorphous cytoplasm without cell borders, nuclei that are multiple and diverse in size and shape, and a continuous syncytial lining. This configuration aids transport.

After implantation is complete, trophoblasts further differentiate along two main pathways, giving rise to villous and extravillous trophoblasts. *Villous trophoblasts* generate chorionic villi, which primarily transport oxygen, nutrients, and other compounds between the fetus and mother. *Extravillous trophoblasts* migrate into the decidua and myometrium and also penetrate maternal vasculature, thus coming into contact with various maternal cell types. Extravillous trophoblasts are further classified as *interstitial trophoblasts* and *endovascular trophoblasts*. The interstitial trophoblasts invade the decidua and eventually penetrate the myometrium to form placental-bed giant cells. These trophoblasts also surround spiral arteries. The endovascular trophoblasts penetrate the spiral artery lumens.

Dermatology

1. Infectious cause of erythema multiforme in given image is:

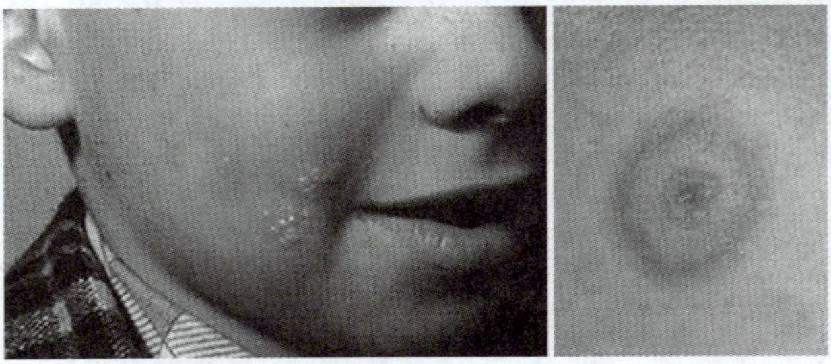

a. Staphylococcus
b. TB
c. HSV
d. EBV

Ans. c. Herpes simplex virus (HSV)

Herpes simplex is the primary cause of erythema multiforme, and the virus is present in 70% of recurrent erythema multiforme cases. Both types of herpes simplex virus (HSV) can cause the condition, but HSV-1, which also causes cold sores, is responsible for most cases.

Causes of Erythema Multiforme

- Idiopathic → Most common cause
- Viral → HSV (most important), HBV, Mumps, Adenovirus
- Bacteria → Streptococci, tuberculosis
- Fungal → Coccidioidomycosis, Histoplasmosis.
- Drugs → Antibiotics (Sulphonamide), Phenytoin, NSAIDs.
- Autoimmune disease → SLE, thyroiditis, RA
- Others → Sarcoidosis, Pregnancy, Malignancy.

2. A young HIV patient with recurrent lesions over genitals as shown in the image. What is the expected microscopic finding in this lesion?

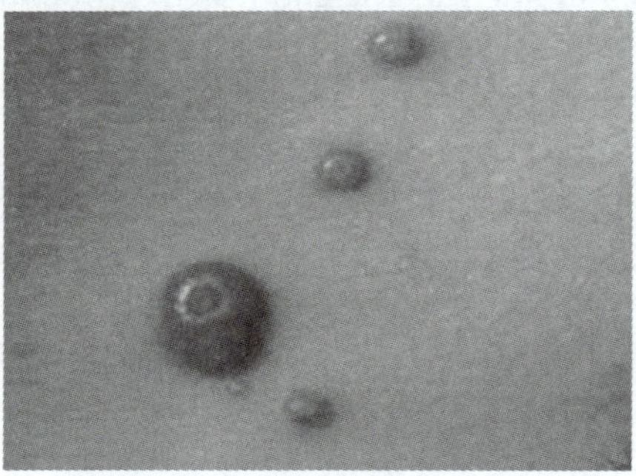

a. Intracytoplasmic inclusion body
b. Intranuclear inclusion body
c. Bacteria with bipolar staining
d. Multinucleated giant cells

Ans. a. Intracytoplasmic inclusion body

Molluscum Contagiosum

Two forms of infection are seen: Childhood variety which is spread by skin-skin contact, and adult variety, which spreads by sexual contact.

- Typical lesion is a pearly, white umbilicated papule from which a white core can be extruded.

Site

- Intertriginous sites such as axillae, popliteal fossa and groin are involved in adults.
- Face is most commonly involved in children

Etiology

- It is caused by molluscum contagiosum virus (MCV), mostly by genotype 1

Histopathology

- Cup shaped thickening of epidermis with characteristic degenerative changes seen in stratum granulosum.
- Basal layer remains intact, above which enlarged cells containing large intracytoplasmic inclusions (Henderson-Paterson bodies) are seen

Treatment

- Spontaneously resolve after squeezing, curettage, cautery and salicylic acid application.
- Topical cantharidin, cidofovir, podophyllin
- Cryotherapy with liquid nitrogen.

3. Patch test read after:

a. 24 and 48 hrs
b. 24 and 72 hrs
c. 48 and 96 hrs
d. 48 and 72 hrs

Ans. c. 48 and 96 hrs

Patch Test

- Patch tests are useful in finding the cause of allergic but not irritant dermatitis. They detect allergens responsible for type IV hypersensitivity.

Closed Patch Test

- Antigens, in standardized dilutions are applied to the back and occluded.

- Adhesive bandage is removed after 48 hours (2 days) for initial interpretation
- Second reading is taken at 96 hours (4 days) to detect delayed reactions.

Open Patch Test

- Allergen is applied on outer arm skin and left uncovered

4. Topical steroids are most effective in:

a. Dermal atrophy b. Eczematous atopic dermatitis
c. Bullous lesions due to HSV d. Nodular acne

Ans. b. Eczematous atopic dermatitis

Atopic Dermatitis (AD)

- It is a type of endogenous eczema triggered by exogenous agents.
- Lesion are extremely pruritic, recurrent, symmetric.
- Family history of atopy is present and the condition usually starts in childhood
- Clinical features vary depending upon the age
  - Infantile phase—Intensely itchy papules and vesicles, starting on the face, but can involve any part of the body except the diaper area.
  - Childhood phase—leathery, itchy plaques mainly on the elbow and knee flexors. Often a reversed extensor pattern is seen.
  - Adult phase—itchy, lichenified plaques, involving the cubital and popliteal fossae.
- Differential diagnosis include contact dermatitis, psoriasis, and seborrheic dermatitis.
- Criteria for diagnosing atopic dermatitis includes one mandatory and five major criteria
- Mandatory criteria includes evidence of pruritic skin, including the report by a parent of a child rubbing or scratching.

In addition to itchy skin, three or more of the following are needed to make the diagnosis:

- History of skin creases being involved. These include: antecubital fossae, popliteal fossae, neck, areas around eyes, fronts of ankles.
- History of asthma or hay fever (or history of atopic disease in a first-degree relative for children <4 years of age).
- The presence of generally dry skin within the past year.
- Symptoms beginning in a child before the age of two years. This criterion is not used to make the diagnosis in a child who is under four years old.
- Visible dermatitis involving flexural surfaces. For children under four years of age, this criterion is met by dermatitis affecting the cheeks or forehead and outer aspects of the extremities.
- *Treatment*: Topical steroids along with oral antihistaminics form the mainstay of therapy.

5. Which of the following cells is not present in the layer of epidermis shown below?

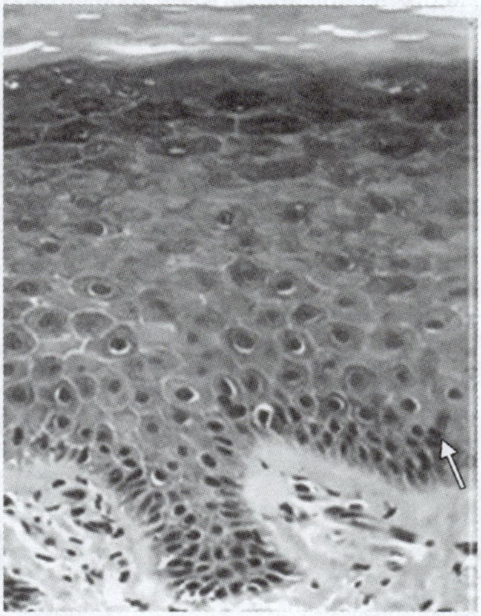

a. Keratinocyte
b. Merkel cell
c. Melanocyte
d. Langerhans cell

Ans. d. Langerhans cell

Layers of Epidermis

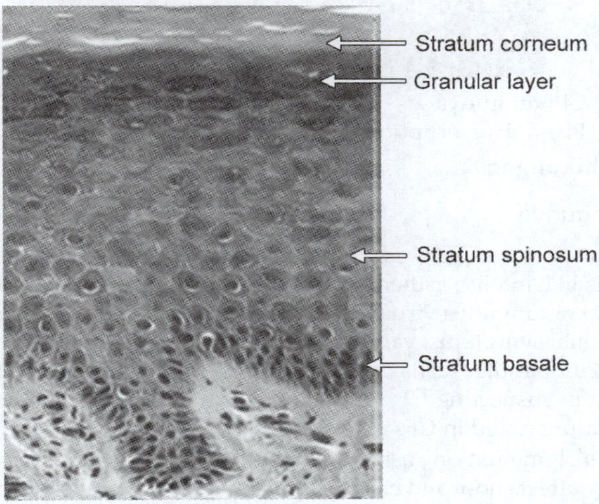

- *Basal layer/stratum germinativum*: Mitotically active keratinocytes. Melanocytes exist admixed with keratinocytes in the basal layer of the epidermis. Merkel cells are sensory receptors present in this layer.
- *Stratum spinosum*: Spines of keratinocytes have abundant desmosomes, Ca^{2+} dependent cell surface modification that promote adhesion of epidermal cells resistance to mechanical stress. Langerhans cells are antigen presenting cells which are most abundant in this layer.
- *Granular layer*: Cells have basophilic keratinohyaline granules composed of profilaggrin keratin filament, loricrin.
- *Stratum corneum*: Layer made of keratin
  - *Corneocyte*: Largest cell of epidermis.
  - Filaggrin responsible for keratin filament aggregation.

6. A patient presented with fever and joint pain for which he was put on NSAIDs. After 10 days the patient developed the following skin lesion. What is the cause for pigmentation?

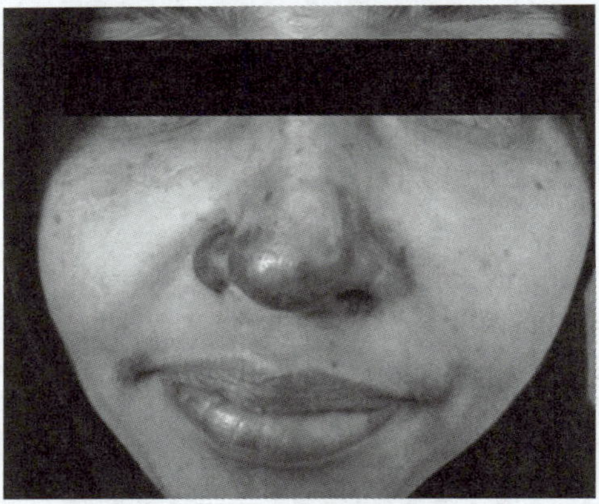

a. Chikungunya b. Dengue
c. Fixed drug eruption d. Melasma

Ans. **a. Chikungunya**

Chikungunya

Chikungunya fever (CF) is an acute febrile illness presenting with symptoms like intense asthenia, arthralgia, myalgia and headache and is caused by chikungunya virus (CV). Apart from fever, joint pain and other constitutional symptoms, various mucocutaneous changes also occur. Of these, maculopapular rash is common in several viral illnesses, therefore, not useful in suspecting CF. On the other hand, hyperpigmentation is a unique feature noted in CF.

Hyperpigmentation associated with CF is macular and most commonly affects nose and cheeks. It may develop soon after the rash has resolved, and has an acute onset. Usually pigmentary changes develop after two weeks or more after the rash; by the time fever has subsided; hence it may be termed as post chikungunya pigmentation (PCP). PCP may occur in the form of discrete macules, freckle-like, diffuse, flagellate, Addisonian type of palmar pigmentation, periorbital melanosis and pigmentation of pre-existing acne lesions.

Involvement of centrofacial face (nose and cheeks) mimics melasma and in a busy outpatient department (OPD), is likely to be missed especially if proper history is not taken. Patients with PCP give a history of high grade fever 2–4 weeks before onset, acute onset of hypermelanosis and many times, persistent asthenia and joint pain even after defervescence of fever.

7. Arrange the following vesiculobullous disorders, based on the epidermal layer involved, in order from superficial to deep:

a. Pemphigus vulgaris
b. Linear IgA disease
c. Pemphigus foliaceous
d. Epidermolysis bullosa dystrophica

Ans. **c. Pemphigus foliaceous, a. Pemphigus vulgaris, b. Linear IgA disease, d. Epidermolysis bullosa dystrophica**

The layer of split in various bullous disorders are summarised in the following image:

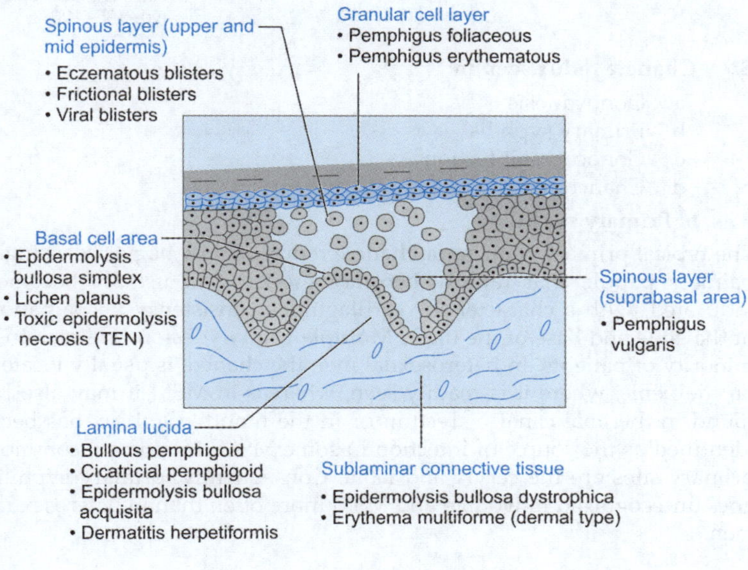

Vesiculo-bullous Disorders

Immunologically mediated bullous disorders				
Disease	Pemphigus vulgaris	Bullous pemphigoid	Linear IgA disease	Dermatitis herpetiformis
Auto antigen	Desmoglein 1, 3	BP230, BP180	BPAg2	Epidermal and tissue transglutaminase
Clinical features	Flaccid blister denuded skin, oral lesions	Large tense blisters on flexor surfaces and trunk	Pruritic small papules on extensor surfaces occasionally larger acneiform blister in adults	Extremely pruritic small vesicles on elbows, knees buttocks and posterior neck
Direct immunofluorescence microscopy	Cells surface deposits of IgG & C3 on keratinocytes in fishnet pattern	Linear band of IgG and /or C3 in epidermal basement membrane	Linear band of IgA, in epidermal basement membrane	Granular deposits of IgA in dermal papillae
Histology	Epidermal acantholytic blister in stratum spinosum (suprabasal layer)	Subepidermal blister with an eosinophil rich infiltrate in perivascular and vesicular sites	Subepidermal blister with neutrophils in dermal papillae	Subepidermal blister with neutrophils in dermal papillae
Associations	HLA-DR4 and DRW6	HLA-DQ	HLA B8 (+) TNF2 allele	Subclinical gluten sensitive enteropathy 100%) HLA-B8 (60%)/ DRW (95%) and HLA–DQW2 haplotype (95–100%)

8. Chancre redux seen in:

a. Donovanosis
b. Primary syphilis
c. Gonococcal infection
d. Chancroid

Ans. b. Primary syphilis

The typical primary chancre or chancre redux usually begins as a single painless papule that rapidly becomes eroded and usually becomes indurated, with a characteristic cartilaginous consistency on palpation of the edge and base of the ulcer. Multiple primary lesions are seen in a minority of patients. In heterosexual men the chancre is usually located on the penis, where it is readily seen, whereas in MSM it may also be found in the anal canal or rectum or in the mouth. Oral sex has been identified as the source of infection in some MSM. In women, common primary sites are the cervix and labia. Consequently, primary syphilis goes unrecognized in women and MSM more often than in heterosexual men.

Major manifestations of various stages of syphilis have been summarized below:

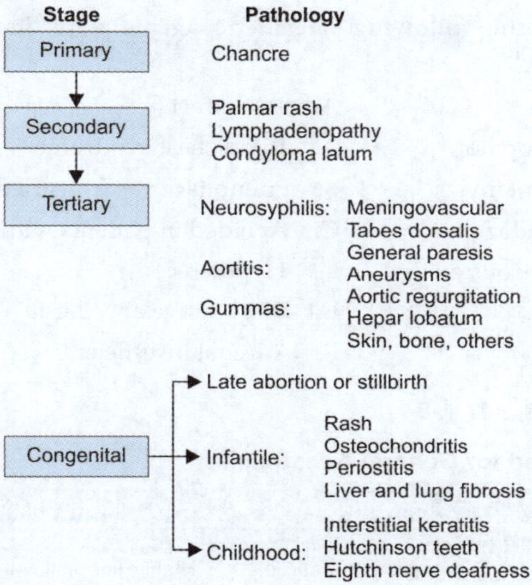

Anesthesia

1. Match the following anesthetic agents with its appropriate property:

Drug	**Adverse effect**
1. Propofol	A. Rigid chest syndrome
2. Fentanyl	B. Pulmonary vasoconstriction
3. Midazolam	C. Avoided in patients with egg allergy
4. Nitrous oxide	D. Hypotension
	E. Dissociative anesthesia
	F. Adrenal insufficiency

Ans. 1-C, 2-A, 3-D, 4-B

Drugs Used for General Anesthesia

Drugs	Therapeutic uses	Clinical pharmacology
Parenteral anesthetics		
Propofol Etomidate Ketamine Thiopental	Anesthetic induction Rapid-onset and short-duration anesthetics used in procedures for rapid return to preoperative mental status	Highly lipophilic → entry to brain and spinal cord, accumulation in fatty tissues **Propofol dosage**: ↓ in elderly due to reduced clearance, ↑ in young children due to rapid clearance, avoided in patients with egg allergy **Etomidate**: preferred for patients at risk of hypotension or MI; produces hypnosis, no analgesic effects, associated with seizures **Ketamine**: suited for patients at risk for hypotension and asthma and for pediatric procedures; increases HR, BP, CO, CBF, and ICP; emergence delirium, hallucinations, vivid dreams, limit use
Barbiturates Methohexital Thiopental	Anesthetic induction	Respiratory and EEG depressants **Methohexital**: more rapid clearance than other barbiturates **Thiopental**: action terminated by redistribution Intra-arterial injection of thiobarbiturates → severe inflammatory and potentially necrotic reaction

Contd...

Contd...

Drugs	Therapeutic uses	Clinical pharmacology
Inhalational anesthetics		
Isoflurane	Maintenance of anesthesia Commonly used inhalational anesthetic	Highly volatile at RT; not flammable in air or O_2 ↓ ventilation and RBF; ↑ CBF Induces hypotension and ↑ coronary blood flow, thus ↓ myocardial O_2 consumption ↓ Baroreceptor function Excreted unchanged by the lungs
Enflurane	Maintenance of anesthesia	Volatile at RT; store in tightly sealed bottles Slow induction and recovery ↓ arterial BP due to vasodilation and ↓ myocardial contractility Possible effects: ↑ ICP, seizure activity
Sevoflurane	Preferred agent for anesthetic induction Used for outpatient anesthesia (not irritating airway; induction and recovery are rapid)	Reacts exothermically with desiccated CO_2 absorbent Ideal induction agent (pleasant smell, rapid onset) ↓AP pressure and CO; potent bronchodilator Preferred for patients with myocardial ischemia Compound A, product of interaction of sevoflurane with the CO_2-absorbent soda lime, is nephrotoxic
Desflurane	Used for outpatient surgery (rapid onset, rapid recovery)	Highly volatile at RT; store in tightly sealed bottles Nonflammable in mixtures of air or O_2 An airway irritant
Halothane	Maintenance of anesthesia	Highly volatile at RT, light sensitive; store in tightly sealed amber bottles with thymol (preservative) Possible hepatic toxicity
Nitrous oxide (N_2O)	Weak anesthetic agent used for its significant analgesic effects	Colorless and odorless gas; used as adjunct to other anesthetics. Will expand volume of air-containing cavities; thus, avoid use in obstructions of ear and bowel, and in intraocular and intracranial air bubbles, etc. To avoid diffusional hypoxia, administer 100% O_2 rather than air when discontinuing N_2O Can increase CBF and ICP, produce vasoconstriction Clinical use of N_2O is controversial due to potential metabolic effects related to increased homocysteine and changes in DNA and protein synthesis
Xenon	Analgesic and anesthetic effects	Rapid induction and emergence from anesthesia In CNS: NMDA receptor antagonist, TREK channel agonist Well tolerated in older patients

Contd...

Contd...

Drugs	Therapeutic uses	Clinical pharmacology
Anesthetic adjuncts augment anesthetic effects of general anesthesia		
Benzodiazepines Midazolam, diazepam, lorazepam	Used for anxiolysis, amnesia, preanesthetic sedation, and sedation during procedures not requiring general anesthesia	Midazolam most commonly used, followed distantly by diazepam and lorazepam; high doses cause respiratory and cardiac depression
α_2 Adrenergic agonists Dexmedetomidine	Short-term (<24 h) sedation of critically ill adults Sedation prior to and during surgical or medical procedures in nonintubated patients	Activation of the α_{2A} adrenergic receptor by dexmedetomidine → sedation and analgesia Side effects: hypotension and bradycardia due to decreased catecholamine release in the CNS; nausea and dry mouth
Analgesics *Opioids* Fentanyl, Sufentanil, Alfentanil, Remifentanil, Meperidine, Morphine	To reduce anesthetic requirement and minimize hemodynamic changes due to painful stimuli	Opioids are the primary analgesics during perioperative period; the choice of opioid is based on duration of action Opioids often are administered intrathecally and epidurally for management of acute and chronic pain Rigid chest syndrome is a rare complication

2. Which is not an advantage of high pressure oxygen administration through nasal cannula?

a. Humidification
b. Bypassing nasopharyngeal dead space
c. PEEP
d. Decreased need for intubation

Ans. b. Bypassing nasopharyngeal dead space

High Flow Nasal Cannula (HFNC)

Supplemental oxygen via nasal cannula and face-masks often is insufficient for patients in severe respiratory distress. Oxygen delivered through a high-flow nasal cannula (HFNC) provides humidified, heated oxygen at flow rates up to 60 L/minute, providing positive pressure and decreasing the work of breathing. HFNC helps in patients with hypoxemia and an intact respiratory drive, often as an alternative to intubation or noninvasive positive-pressure ventilation. It is best avoided in those not breathing or with bullous lung disease and pneumothoraces. Another option is flush rate oxygenation, where the wall oxygen unit is turned past 15 L/minutes to maximum flow rates of 40–60 L/minute. The latter aids avoiding desaturation during rapid intubation techniques in addition to other respiratory distress events. Both HFNC and flush rate oxygenation are best seen as bridges to awaiting clinical improvement or other ventilation methods. Nasal prongs, however, do not bypass the nasopharyngeal dead space unlike endotracheal intubation.

3. Duration of action of proparacaine:

a. 2 min b. 5 min
c. 10 min d. 20 min

Ans. c. 10 min

Topical Anesthetics Used in Ophthalmology

Topical anesthetics are useful for diagnostic and therapeutic procedures, including tonometry, removal of foreign bodies or sutures, gonioscopy, corneal or conjunctival scraping, and minor surgical operations on the cornea and conjunctiva. Cataract (phacoemulsification) surgery is increasingly being carried out under topical anesthesia, supplemented if necessary by (intracameral) injection of local anesthetic into the anterior chamber or oral or intravenous sedation.

Proparacaine, tetracaine, and benoxinate are the most commonly used topical anesthetics. For practical purposes, they can be said to have equivalent anesthetic potency.

Benoxinate Hydrochloride

- *Preparation*: Solution, 0.4% combined with 0.25% fluorescein sodium
- *Dosage:* 1 drop and repeat as necessary.
- *Onset and duration of action:* Anesthesia begins within 1 or 2 minutes and lasts for 10–15 minutes.

Proparacaine Hydrochloride (Proxymetacaine)

- *Preparations:* Solution, 0.5%; 0.5% combined with 0.25% fluorescein (Fluoracaine).
- *Dosage:* 1 drop and repeat as necessary.
- *Onset and duration of action:* Anesthesia begins within 20 seconds and lasts 10–15 minutes.
- *Comment:* Least irritating of the topical anesthetics and most suitable for corneal scraping for microbiological cultures.

Tetracaine Hydrochloride (Pontocaine)

- *Preparation:* Solution, 0.5%
- *Dosage:* 1 drop and repeat as necessary.
- *Onset and duration of action:* Anesthesia occurs within 1 minute and lasts for 15–20 minutes.
- *Comment:* Stings considerably on instillation.

Radiology

1. Image of FAST. What is the inference?

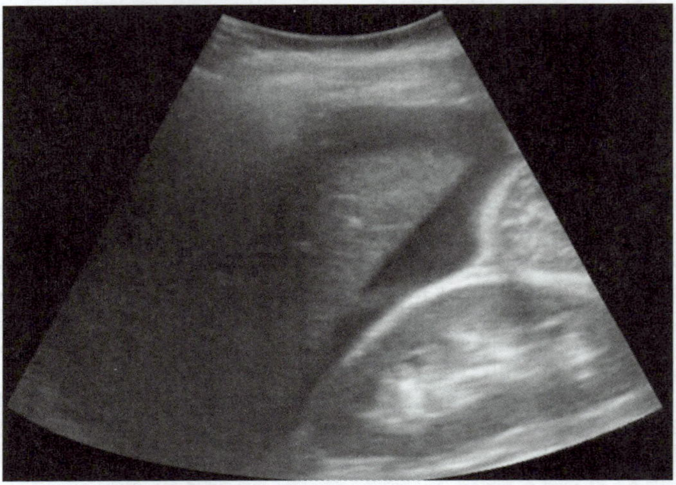

a. FAST positive
b. FAST negative
c. FAST inconclusive
d. FAST

Ans. a. FAST positive

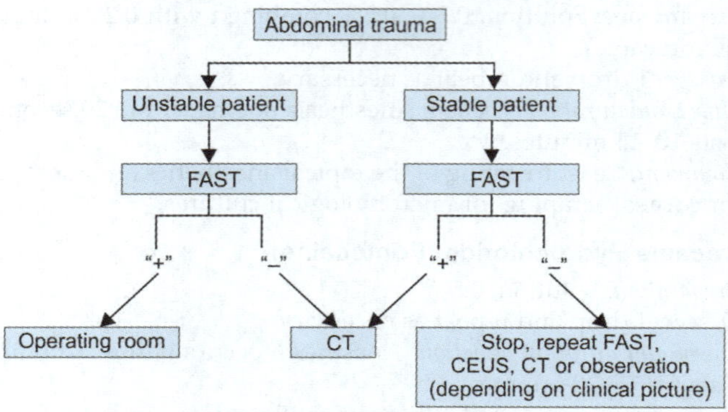

FAST: focused assessment with sonography for trauma;
CT: computed tomography.

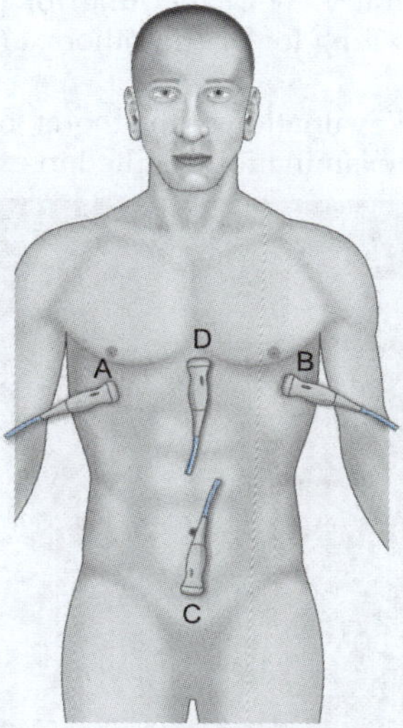

The original FAST scan included views of (A) the right upper quadrant, which included the perihepatic area and hepatorenal recess or Morison pouch; (B) the left upper quadrant, encompassing the perisplenic view; (C) the suprapubic view (pouch of Douglas), and later; (D) a subxiphoid pericardial view

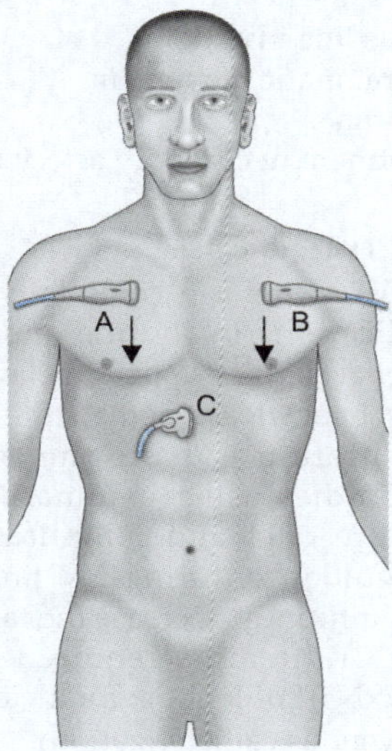

(A) right parasagittal view of the lung for pneumothorax; (B) left parasagittal view of the lung for pneumothorax; (C) a longitudinal view of the IVC.

The addition of US evaluation of the thorax to detect pneumothorax to the traditional FAST examination resulted in extended FAST (eFAST)

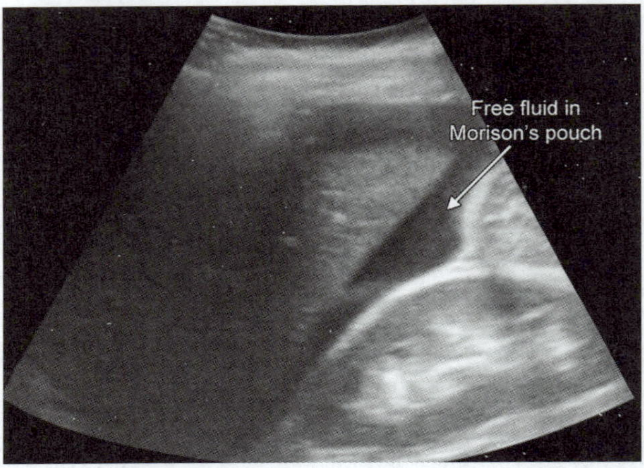

In the image given in the question, anechoic fluid is seen between the liver and kidney (the hepatorenal pouch of Morison), which is suggestive of hemoperitoneum in a trauma setting.

2. Utility of USG (true/false):

a. Central venous line insertion
b. Assess diaphragmatic movement
c. Useful in trauma
d. Useful in treatment of coronary artery disease
e. None

Ans. a. True, b. True, c. True, d. False

a. Central venous (CV) access is a commonly performed procedure with multiple indications in routine and emergent situations. Access to the internal jugular vein, subclavian vein, and femoral vein has typically been described in the emergency medicine and critical care literature using the traditional landmark-based approach. Studies using landmark-based methods have reported high failure rates and complication rates. The use of ultrasonographic guidance during CV line placement has been demonstrated to significantly decrease the failure rate, complication rate, and number of attempts required for successful access https://youtu.be/rWxN4JFBEJc (Link for a video showing how USG is useful in central venous catheterization)

b. The diagnostic tools traditionally used to study diaphragm dysfunction, such as fluoroscopy, phrenic nerve conduction study, and transdiaphragmatic pressure measurement, present some limitations and disadvantages, including the use of ionizing radiation, low availability, invasiveness, and the need for patient transportation and skilled or specifically trained operators. Recently, ultrasound has been used to evaluate diaphragmatic function. Advantages of ultrasound include safety, avoidance of radiation hazards, and availability at the bedside. Diaphragmatic displacement is measured using ultrasound as a measure of diaphragmatic function.
c. Focused assessment with sonography for Trauma (FAST) rapidly assesses for hemoperitoneum and hemopericardium, and the Extended FAST examination (EFAST) explores for hemothorax, pneumothorax and intravascular filling status. In regional trauma, ultrasound can be used to detect fractures, many vascular injuries, musculoskeletal injuries, testicular injuries and can assess fetal viability in pregnant trauma patients. Ultrasound can also be used at the bedside to guide procedures in trauma, including nerve blocks and vascular access. Importantly, these examinations are being performed by the treating physician in real time, allowing for immediate changes to management of the patient.
d. There is no established use of ultrasound in treatment of coronary artery disease. Stenting is performed for symptomatic coronary artery occlusion and is done using Digital Subtraction Angiography (DSA), not ultrasound.

3. In which of the lung pathologies, MRI is preferred over CT?

a. Pulmonary embolism
b. Tuberculosis
c. Pancoast tumor
d. Pleural effusion

Ans. c. Pancoast tumor

In most of the lung pathologies CT is the modality of choice

- *HRCT*: High resolution CT consists of very thin high resolution sections with some gap in between the slices. It is the modality of choice for diffuse lung disease where the disease process involves the entire/bulk of the lung fields but need detailed inspection of the lung parenchyma e.g. interstitial lung diseases.
- *CECT*: It is used to see the contrast characteristics of the lesions like lung nodules/masses, mediastinal lymph nodes (central non-enhancement seen in necrotic nodes in tuberculosis), vascular pathologies.
- *MRI*: It is not commonly used in lung pathologies but one of the important indications is Pancoast tumors (tumors involving the lung apices).

As these tumors tend to involve the nerves of the brachial plexus and MRI is the modality of choice for looking at nervous tissue, thus in pancoast tumors MRI is preferred over CT.

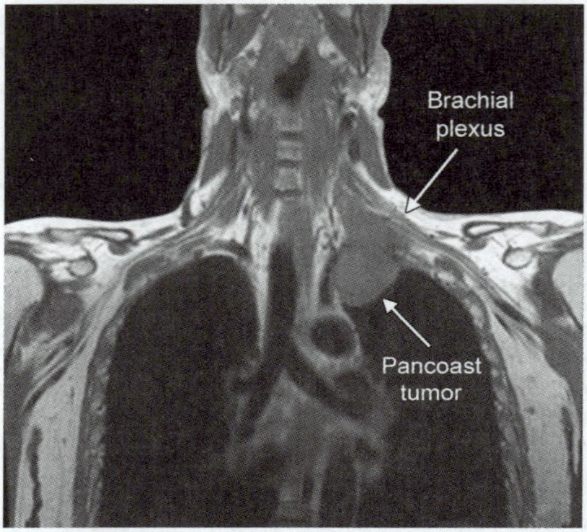

Chest magnetic resonance imaging of a left pancoast tumor arising in the left upper lobe and infiltrating the first rib, brachial plexus.

4. Assertion/Reason:

Assertion: Investigation of choice for aortic dissection is MDCT
Reason: In experienced hands transthoracic echo is as sensitive and specific for detecting dissection as MDCT

a. Both Assertion and Reasoning are independently true/correct and Reason is the correct explanation of the Assertion
b. Both Assertion and Reasoning are independently true/correct and Reason is not the correct explanation of the Assertion
c. Assertion is independently a true/correct statement but the Reason is independently an incorrect/false statement
d. Assertion is independently a false/incorrect statement but the Reason is independently a true/correct statement
e. Both Assertion and Reason are independently a false/incorrect statement

Ans. b. Both Assertion and Reasoning are independently true/correct and Reason is not the correct explanation of the Assertion
Aortic dissection is the most common form of the acute aortic syndromes and a type of arterial dissection. It occurs when blood enters the medial

layer of the aortic wall through a tear or penetrating ulcer in the intima and tracks along the media, forming a second blood-filled channel within the wall.

The normal lumen lined by intima is called the *true lumen* and the blood-filled channel in the media is called the *false lumen*. In most cases the vessel wall is abnormal. Causes include:

- Hypertension (pathogenesis: medial degeneration)
- Inherited connective tissue disorders (pathogenesis: medial degeneration)
  - Marfan syndrome
  - Ehlers-Danlos syndrome
- Atherosclerosis (pathogenesis: penetrating ulcer)
- Vasculitis (pathogenesis: inflammation)

Imaging is essential in delineating the morphology and extent of the dissection as well as allowing for classification (which dictates management). Two classification systems are in common usage, both of which divide dissections according to the involvement of the ascending aorta:

1. Stanford classification (Preferred nowadays)
2. DeBakey classification

CT, especially with arterial contrast enhancement (CTA) is the investigation of choice, able not only to diagnose and classify the dissection but also to evaluate for distal complications. It has reported sensitivity and specificity of nearly 100%.

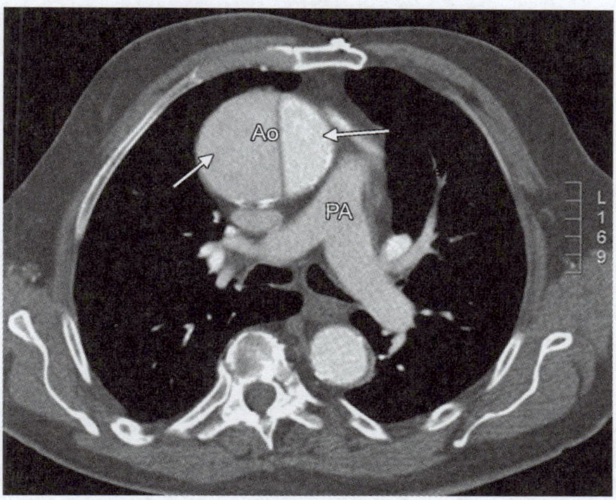

True lumen	False lumen
Often compressed by the false lumen and the smaller of the two	Often larger lumen size due to higher false luminal pressures
Origin of celiac trunk, SMA and right renal artery usually from true lumen	At risk for rupture due to reduced elastic recoil and dilation
Outer wall calcifications (helpful in acute dissections)	Often of lower contrast density due to delayed opacification
	Origin of left renal artery usually from false lumen

Transesophageal echocardiography (TOE) has very high sensitivity and specificity for assessment of acute aortic dissection, but due to limited access and its invasive nature, it has largely been replaced by CTA (or MRA in some instances)

Educational objective: Both the statements are correct. But the two statements are not related to each other. The reason for MDCT being the investigation of choice is that it is non-invasive, easily available and highly sensitive and specific.

Psychiatry

1. Paradoxical suicide refers to:

a. Suicide during recovery of illness
b. Accidental suicide
c. Suicide on low dose of drug
d. Failed attempt to suicide

Ans. a. Suicide during recovery of illness

In some psychiatric disorders, most commonly in depression, there is an increased incidence of suicides during recovery of the illness. Major depressive episodes can be precipitated by a variety of mechanisms, including the administration of medications. Multiple cases have been reported in which antidepressant medication appeared to exacerbate a major depressive episode to the point of suicide. Subsequent withdrawal of the initial medication led to a partial remission in each case and points out the possibility of antidepressant medication precipitating suicidal behavior and underscores the need for careful monitoring of symptomatology.

2. All are true for depersonalisation *except*:

a. More common in females than males
b. Common in patients with seizure and migraine
c. Common after life threatening accidents
d. Reality testing is deranged during the episode

Ans. d. Reality testing is deranged during the episode

Depersonalization/Derealization Disorder

Clinical Findings

Depersonalization/derealization disorder is defined as the presence of persistent or recurrent experiences of depersonalization, derealization or both. It is more common in females and can occur after emotional trauma. Depersonalization is defined as experiences of unreality, detachment or being an outside observer with respect to one's thoughts, feelings, sensations, body or actions (e.g., perceptual alterations, distorted sense of time, unreal or absent self, emotional and/or physical numbing). Derealization is defined as experiences of unreality or detachment with respect to surroundings (e.g., individuals or objects are experienced as unreal, dream-like, foggy, lifeless or visually distorted). During the depersonalization or derealization experiences, reality testing remains intact. This means that the person has the awareness that it is only a feeling and not a reality.

The onset is usually sudden and typically occurs in a setting of anxiety. Patients feel numb and out of touch with their feelings, bodies, and surroundings. Sometimes they feel as if they are observing themselves or as though they are automations in a dream. Depersonalization is difficult to describe, and patients may express concern about "going crazy," particularly if the condition is accompanied by déjà vu experiences and distortions in the sense of time. Depression and anxiety are commonly associated with depersonalization.

Associated Conditions

Depersonalization is likely to be elicited from patients with anxiety disorders (particularly panic disorder), other dissociative disorders, depressive disorder, and borderline personality disorder. Depersonalization has been reported in 11–42% of schizophrenic patients. In schizophrenia, depersonalization tends to become incorporated into the prevailing delusional system. Depersonalization may also be encountered in substance abuse, particularly with alcohol, marijuana, hallucinogens, cocaine, phenylcyclidine, methylamphetamine, narcotics, and sedatives. Depersonalization has also been reported after medication with indomethacin, fenfluramine, and haloperidol.

Migraine and seizures are the most common conditions associated with depersonalization. In epilepsy, particularly temporal lobe epilepsy, depersonalization may be encountered as an aura, as part of the seizure itself, or between seizures. Depersonalization in epilepsy is more likely to be associated with stereotypic movements (e.g., lip smacking), senseless words or phrases, and loss of consciousness than in dissociative disorders, in which it is likely to be more highly elaborated. Depersonalization may also be evident in postconcussive disorder, Meniere disease, cerebral atherosclerosis, and Korsakoff syndrome.

Treatment

If depersonalization is a subsidiary symptom, the primary disorder should be treated. There have been no controlled studies of treatment for depersonalization disorder proper. The relative effectiveness of supportive psychotherapy, hypnosis, exploratory psychotherapy, family therapy, and cognitive–behavioral therapy is not known. Psychotherapy focuses on the recovery of the traumatic experience from which the pathologic dissociation is thought to have arisen. Hypnosis may help in this regard. Cognitive–behavioral desensitization, flooding, and exposure have also been used.

3. True about grades of insight, *except*:

a. Grade 1—complete denial of illness
b. Grade 2—slight awareness of being sick and needing help but denying it at the same time
c. Grade 3—awareness of being sick, due to something unknown in self
d. Grade 6—true emotional insight

Ans. c. Grade 3—awareness of being sick, due to something unknown in self

Insight

The assessment of insight in people with schizophrenia and other psychiatric illness is an important part of the mental status examination. Insight is defined as "A person's capacity to understand the nature, significance and severity of his or her own illness."

Grades of insight include:

1. Complete denial of illness
2. Slight awareness of being sick and needing help but denying it at the same time.
3. Awareness of being sick but blaming it on others, external factors, or medical or unknown organic factors.
4. Awareness of being sick, due to something unknown in self
5. *Intellectual insight*: Admission of illness and recognition that symptoms or failures in social adjustment are due to irrational feelings or disturbances, without applying that knowledge to future experiences.
6. *True emotional insight*: Emotional awareness of the motives and feelings within and of the underlying meaning of symptoms, whether the awareness leads to changes in personality, and future behavior; openness to new ideas and concepts about self and important people in the person's life.

Pediatrics

1. Assertion: Antibiotics should not be given to children having diarrhea:

Reason: Diarrhea in children is mostly caused by viruses

a. Both Assertion and Reasoning are independently true/correct and Reason is the correct explanation of the Assertion

b. Both Assertion and Reasoning are independently true/correct and Reason is not the correct explanation of the Assertion

c. Assertion is independently a true/correct statement but the Reason is independently an incorrect/false statement

d. Assertion is independently a false/incorrect statement but the Reason is independently a true/correct statement

e. Both Assertion and Reason are independently a false/incorrect statement

Ans. **a. Both Assertion and Reasoning are independently true/correct and Reason is the correct explanation of the Assertion**

Acute viral gastroenteritis is the most common cause of vomiting and diarrhea in children and continues to cause approximately 800,000 deaths globally each year in children <5 years old. Transmission of GI infections can be reduced by attention to good hand hygiene. Handwashing can reduce the incidence of diarrheal disease by approximately 30% in both high- and low-income countries. The provision of alcohol-based hand sanitizer and educational materials can reduce GI illnesses in child care centers, and a multifactorial intervention including hand sanitizer and surface disinfection similarly reduces illness due to enteric pathogens in elementary school students.

Viruses are the most common cause of acute gastroenteritis in developing and developed countries. Of the viral agents causing enteric infection, rotavirus, a 67-nm double-stranded RNA virus with at least eight serotypes, is the most commonly identified. As with most viral pathogens, rotavirus affects the small intestine, causing voluminous watery diarrhea without leukocytes or blood. The virus is transmitted via the fecal-oral route and survives for hours on hands and for days on environmental surfaces. The Norwalk agent (now called norovirus), a calicivirus, is a small RNA virus that mainly causes vomiting but can also cause diarrhea in older children and adults, usually in common source outbreaks. The duration of symptoms is short, usually 24–48 hours. Other potentially pathogenic viruses include astroviruses, corona-like viruses, and other small round viruses.

2. A 5-year-old child presents with fever and altered sensorium for 3 days. On examination, he has lesions on his palm as shown in the image. What is most likely causative organism?

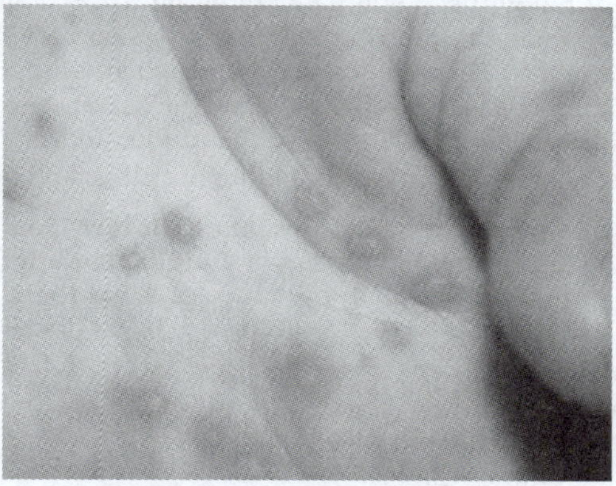

a. Staphylococcus aureus
b. Measles virus
c. Rubella virus
d. Picorna virus

Ans. **d. Picorna virus**

The term Picornaviridae is derived from pico, which means small (typically, 18–30 nm), and RNA, referring to the single-stranded positive-sense RNA common to all members of the Picornaviridae family. All members of this family, whose RNA molecules range from 7.2–8.5 kilobases (kb) in size, lack a lipid envelope and are therefore resistant to ether, chloroform, and alcohol. However, ionizing radiation, phenol, and formaldehyde readily inactivate picorna viruses.

The viral capsid of picorna viruses consists of a densely packed icosahedral arrangement of 60 protomers. Each protomer consists of 4 polypeptides, etoposide (VP) 1, 2, 3, and 4, which all derive from the cleavage of a larger protein. The capsid-coat protein serves multiple functions, including protecting the viral RNA from degradation by environmental RNase, determining host and tissue tropism by recognition of cell-specific cell-membrane receptors, penetrating target cells and delivering the viral RNA into the cell cytoplasm, and selecting and packaging viral RNA.

Two genera of Picornaviridae—enterovirus and rhinovirus—have an identical morphology but can be distinguished based on clinical, biophysical, and epidemiological studies. Enteroviruses grow at a wide pH range (i.e., 3-10). After initial replication in the oropharynx, enteroviruses survive the acidic environment of the stomach. The small intestine is the major invasion site of enteroviruses, which replicate best at 37°C. Rhinoviruses replicate at a pH of 6–8. After initial replication in the nasal passages, the acidic environment of the stomach destroys rhinoviruses. Rhinoviruses optimally replicate at 33°C and primarily infect the nasal mucosa. Infection with various picorna viruses may be asymptomatic or may cause clinical syndromes such as aseptic meningitis (the most common acute viral disease of the CNS), encephalitis, the common cold, febrile rash illnesses (hand-foot-and-mouth disease), conjunctivitis, herpangina, myositis and myocarditis, and hepatitis.

3. A baby, 18 months of age, presents with low grade fever for 3 days. On examination, he has a bulging anterior fontanelle. CSF examination revealed low glucose. What is the most likely diagnosis?

a. Meningitis
b. Pneumonia
c. Intracranial hemorrhage
d. Pseudotumor cerebri

Ans. a. Meningitis

Clinical Features of Meningitis in Children

Neonates and infants <90 days old may have fever, normal temperature, or hypothermia. A normal temperature does exclude meningitis. Toxic appearance, lethargy, mottling, bulging fontanelle, abnormal cry, grunting, respiratory distress, and increased or decreased tone are all supportive of the diagnosis, but these signs can be absent. Jaundice or rash may occasionally be seen. Infants in the first months of life are unlikely to have a stiff neck. Fever in neonates (rectal temperature of 100.5°F or higher) should always prompt suspicion for meningitis. In the absence of fever, a clinician should be concerned about infants who are ill appearing, have the signs or symptoms listed earlier, or are just not "acting right" according to their caregivers.

Older infants (>90 days old) with meningitis may also have fever, hypothermia, toxic appearance, lethargy, mottling, bulging fontanelle, abnormal cry, grunting, and respiratory distress at presentation. Children (>36 months of age) may have fever and nuchal rigidity. The Kernig sign (with the patient lying supine and the hip flexed at 90 degrees, the patient cannot extend the knee fully without pain) and Brudzinski sign (with the patient lying supine, there is involuntary flexion of the legs with passive neck flexion) may be present. Children may have altered mental status, shock, focal neurologic signs, or signs of increased intracranial pressure. Rash or another focal sign of infection may be present. Consider bacterial meningitis in the child with seizures, outside the range of 6 months to 6 years.

CSF Findings in Various Etiologies of Meningitis

Test	Appearance	Pressure	WBC/mL	Protein mg/dL	Glucose mg/dL	Chloride
Normal CSF	Clear	90–180 mm	0–8 lymph	15–45	50–80	115–130 mEq/L
Acute bacterial meningitis	Turbid	Increased	100—10000	100-500	<40	Decreased
Viral meningitis	Clear	Normal to moderate increase	5–300, rarely > 1000	Normal to mild increased	Normal	Normal
Tubercular meningitis	Slightly opaque cobweb formation	Increased/ decreased, spinal block	100–600 mixed or lymph	50–300 due to spinal block	Decreased	Decreased
Fungal meningitis	Clear	Increased	40–400 mixed	50–300	Decreased	Decreased
Acute syphilitic	Clear	Increased	About 500 lymph	Increased but < 100	Normal	Normal

4. Choose the right option among the key words, for the following clinical scenarios:

Theme: Seizure

Key words:

a. Rectal diazepam
b. Inhalation phenobarbitone
c. Intramuscular propofol
d. Intravenous phenytoin
e. Intravenous midazolam
f. Oral valproate
g. Intranasal carbamazepine

Clinical Scenario: 1

A baby was found convulsing for 45 minutes. Senior Resident recommends intravenous lorazepam. Junior Resident could not get intravenous access. Next step in the management is?

Clinical Scenario: 2

When Senior Resident comes back, intravenous access has been established but Baby is still convulsing. What should be the next step?

Ans. **a. Rectal diazepam, e. Intravenous midazolam**

Case 1-Rectal diazepam, Case 2-Intravenous Midazolam

Treatment of status epilepticus in children

Benzodiazepines are the first-line treatment for prolonged seizures because of their rapid onset and effectiveness; however, not all benzodiazepines or routes are available in the prehospital setting, and establishing IV access can be difficult in a child who is having a seizure. Benzodiazepines may be given by the intranasal, buccal, rectal, or intraosseous route when an IV is difficult to place. Rectal diazepam is one "rescue" medication commonly used at home and by EMS personnel. The advantage is that no refrigeration or IV line is needed. The disadvantage is its short half-life and the need for rectal administration. Midazolam, also an effective rescue medication, can be given safely via the intranasal route using a mucosal atomization device. Midazolam can also be given buccally. Lorazepam is not generally used in the prehospital setting because of its need for refrigeration and recommendations that it only be administered through an IV line.

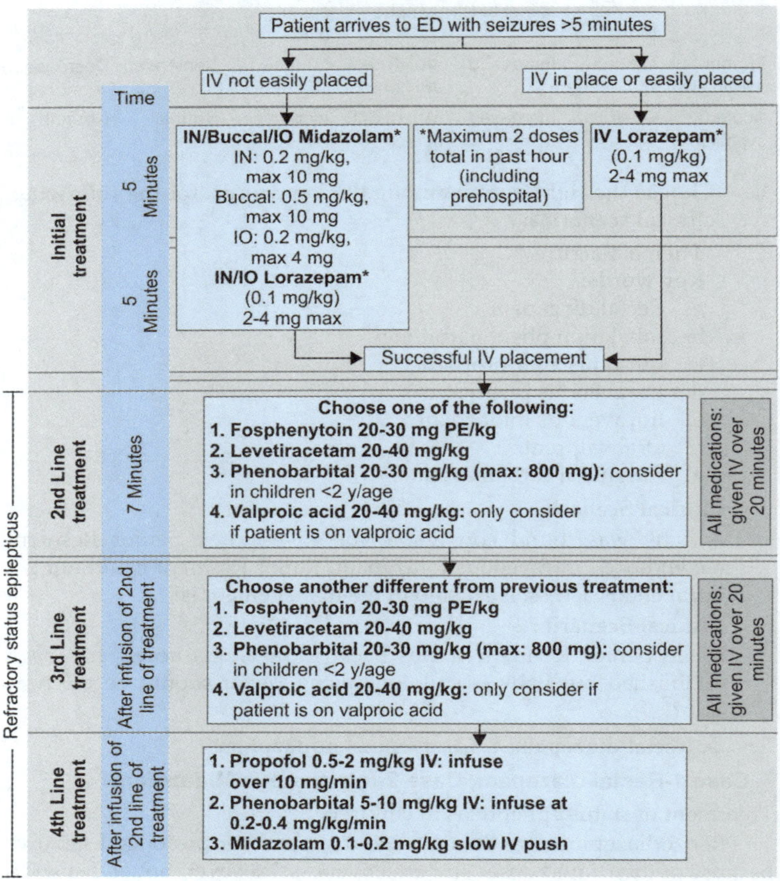

5. A girl of 6 years age can climb up stairs with alternate feet, ride a tricycle, can remember name, age but cannot narrate stories. What is her actual developmental age?

a. 3 years　　b. 4 years
c. 5 years　　d. 6 years

Ans. a. 3 years

Developmental Milestones

Gross Motor

Age	Milestone
3 months	Neck holding
5 months	Rolls over
6 months	Sits in tripod position
8 months	Sits without support
10 months	Stands with support
12 months	Stands without support
15 months	Walks alone
18 months	Runs
2 years	Walks up and downstairs, 2 feet per step
3 years	Rides tricycle, alternate feet going upstairs
4 years	Hops on one foot, alternate feet going downstairs

Fine Motor

Age	Milestone
4 months	Bidextrous approach
6 months	Unidextrous approach
9 months	Immature pincer grasp
12 months	Mature pincer grasp
15 months	Imitates scribbling, tower of 2 blocks, drinks from cup
18 months	Scribbles, tower of 3 blocks, feeds with spoon
2 years	Tower of 6 blocks, verticular and circular strokes, undresses
3 years	Tower of 9 blocks, copies circle, dresses
4 years	Copies cross, bridge with blocks
5 years	Copies triangle, gate with blocks

Social and Adaptive

Age	Milestone
2 months	Social smile
3 months	Recognizes mother
6 months	Stranger anxiety, inhibits to no
9 months	Waves bye bye, repeats activity when appreciated
12 months	Comes when called, plays simple ball game
15 months	Jargon, points to objects of interest
18 months	Copies parents in task

Contd...

Contd...

Age	Milestone
2 years	Asks for food, drink, toilet
3 years	Shares toys, knows full name and gender
4 years	Plays cooperatively in group, goes to toilet alone
5 years	Helps in household tasks

Language

Age	Milestone
1 month	Alerts to sound
3 months	Coos
4 months	Laughs loud
6 months	Monosyllables
9 months	Bisyllables
12 months	1–2 words with meaning
18 months	8–10 word vocabulary
2 years	2–3 word sentences, uses pronouns
3 years	Asks questions
4 years	Sings song, tell stories
5 years	Asks meaning of words

6. Identify the procedure being performed in a baby admitted in NICU as shown in the given images:

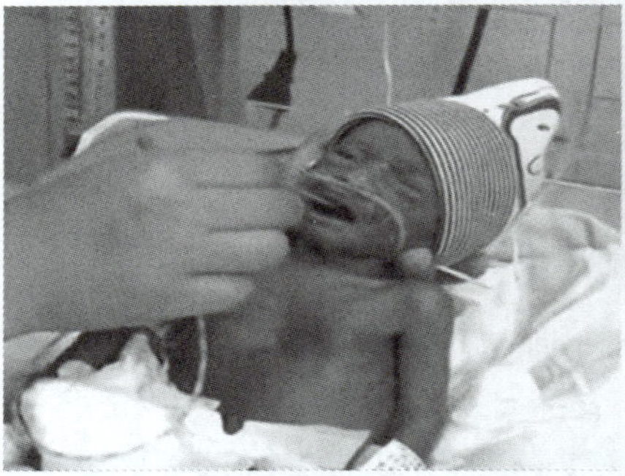

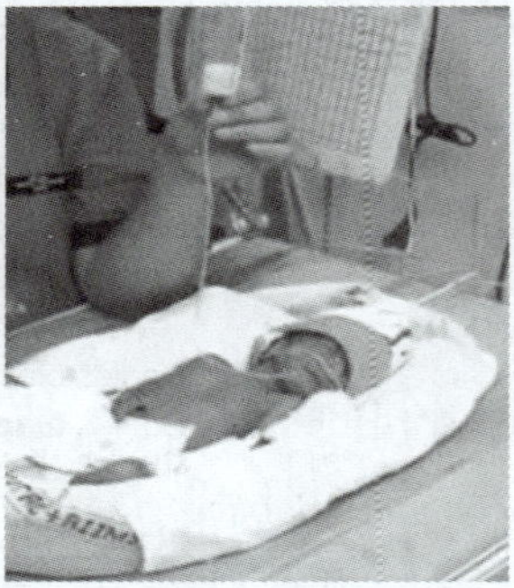

a. Nasogastric feeding
b. Orogastric feeding
c. Orogastric suction
d. Nasopharyngeal suction

Ans. b. Orogastric feeding

The placement and use of gastric tubes are one of the most common nursing procedures performed in the newborn intensive care unit (NICU). These tubes are used for gastric decompression, enteral nutrition and medication administration. Few patients in the NICU will avoid having a gastric tube placed at some point during their hospitalization.

Maturation of oral feeding skills and the choice of initial feeding in low birth weight babies		
Gestational age	***Maturation of feeding skills***	***Initial feeding skills***
< 28 weeks	Inadequate sucking efforts Lack of gut motility	IV fluids
28–31 weeks	Sucking bursts develop Lack of coordination between suck, swallow and breathing	Orogastric or nasogastric feeding
32–34 weeks	Slightly mature sucking pattern Coordination between breathing and swallowing begins	Spoon feeding
> 34 weeks	Mature sucking pattern Coordination between breathing and swallowing	Breastfeeding

7. A lady developed chicken poxduring pregnancy. Highest risk of transmission to fetus is at which period of gestation?

a. 11–14 weeks
b. 14–18 weeks
c. 34–37 weeks
d. 28–32 weeks

Ans. c. 34–37 weeks

Mother to child transmission of varicella causes two distinct types of presentations depending upon the period of gestation. The risk of transmission also depends on the period of gestation— 0.4% in 1st trimester, 2% in 13–20 weeks, 17–30% if onset occurs between 5 days before and 2 days after delivery.

Congenital Varicella Syndrome (Varicella Embryopathy)

Usually results from varicella infection in mother during 8–20 weeks of gestation.

Clinical Manifestations

- *Cicatricial skin lesions*: Cicatrix presenting as a zigzag scarring in a dermatomal distribution
  - Hypopigmentation
- Limb reduction defects and limb hypoplasia – shortened — malformed extremities
- *CNS manifestations*: Microcephaly and cerebral calcification, motor/ sensory deficit, absent deep tendon reflexes, incontinence
- *Ocular manifestations*: Anisocoria, Horner's syndrome.

Investigations

- *Rapid method*: Direct immunofluorescence
- *Confirmatory test*: VZV DNA detection by PCR

Neonatal Varicella

Neonates born to mothers who develop varicella from 5 days before to 2 days after delivery are at high risk for severe or fatal (5%) disease and must be given varicella-zoster immunoglobulin (VariZIG) and followed closely.

8. A three weeks old baby has ambiguous genitalia, BP- 70/45 mm Hg, serum potassium-6 mEq/dL, serum sodium 127 mEq/dL, blood glucose-70 mg%. Patient was started on intravenous fluids. Which of the following specific treatment options will you add?

a. Insulin
b. Potassium exchange resin
c. Hydrocortisone
d. None of the above

Ans. **c. Hydrocortisone**

Congenital Adrenal Hyperplasia

Congenital adrenal hyperplasia results from deficiency in one of the five enzymes involved in the production of cortisol. Absence of these enzymes leads to decreased conversion of 17-hydroxyprogesterone to 11-desoxycortisol with resultant cortisol deficiency. Most of the enzyme deficiencies also impair conversion to progesterone and 11-desoxycorticosterone in the mineralocorticoid pathway, which leads to decreased aldosterone production. Deficiency of 21-hydroxylase accounts for up to 95% of congenital adrenal hyperplasia cases. Seventy-five percent of affected newborns manifest the classic salt-losing, virilizing variant in which urinary salt wasting with hyperkalemia and hyponatremia dominate the clinical picture. Twenty-five percent of cases are the non–salt-losing simple virilizing type. Infants with salt-losing forms of congenital adrenal hyperplasia typically present during the second to fifth weeks of life in crisis, sometimes before the results of newborn screening tests for the disease are available.

Clinical Features

Salt-wasting variants of congenital adrenal hyperplasia typically manifest as acute crisis in the second week of life. Symptoms are vague and include lethargy, irritability, poor feeding, vomiting, and poor weight gain. Depending on the duration and severity of symptoms, infants may present with significant dehydration or even shock. Obtain a complete history of the presenting symptoms, because the differential diagnosis of adrenal salt-wasting crisis includes sepsis, congenital heart disease, and other inborn errors of metabolism. Genitalia: females may have fusion of the labia and an enlarged clitoris. Males may have normal genitalia or a small phallus or hypospadias.

Lab Diagnosis

Although hypoglycemia is rare, poor feeding and vomiting may cause secondary hypoglycemia requiring urgent treatment. The classic electrolyte abnormalities in salt-wasting congenital adrenal hyperplasia are hyponatremia and hyperkalemia. Serum potassium level may be elevated between 6 and 12 mEq/L, although changes in cardiac function and ECG are unusual. Metabolic acidosis typically accompanies the classic electrolyte abnormalities as a result of aldosterone deficiency and dehydration.

Definitive diagnosis depends on analysis of blood hormone levels.

Treatment

Circulatory collapse from cortisol deficiency and dehydration is common, so establish IV or IO access rapidly. Administer IV fluids in the form of 10 to 20 mL/kg of normal saline. Fluid loss in congenital adrenal hyperplasia is isotonic, and fluid replacement should be with normal saline. Treat hypoglycemia with 5 mL/kg of 10% dextrose.

Initiate steroid hormone replacement urgently: give hydrocortisone, 25 milligrams IV/IO to neonates, 50 milligrams to toddlers and school-age children, and 100 milligrams to adolescents. Although mineralocorticoid deficiency in congenital adrenal hyperplasia is primarily treated by sodium repletion with normal saline, there is some mineralocorticoid effect at these doses of hydrocortisone.

If hyperkalemia results in ECG changes or arrhythmia, treat with IV calcium gluconate (10%), 100 milligrams/kg (1 mL/kg), and sodium bicarbonate, 1 mEq/kg. Do not give insulin and glucose for hyperkalemia in infants, because this may result in profound hypoglycemia. The administration of normal saline and hydrocortisone is usually sufficient to lower serum potassium levels in the absence of cardiac manifestations.

9. Effective sign of neonatal resuscitation is:

a. Color change
b. Air entry
c. Heart rate increases
d. None of the above

Ans. **c. Heart rate increaseds**

Neonatal resuscitation algorithm—2015 update

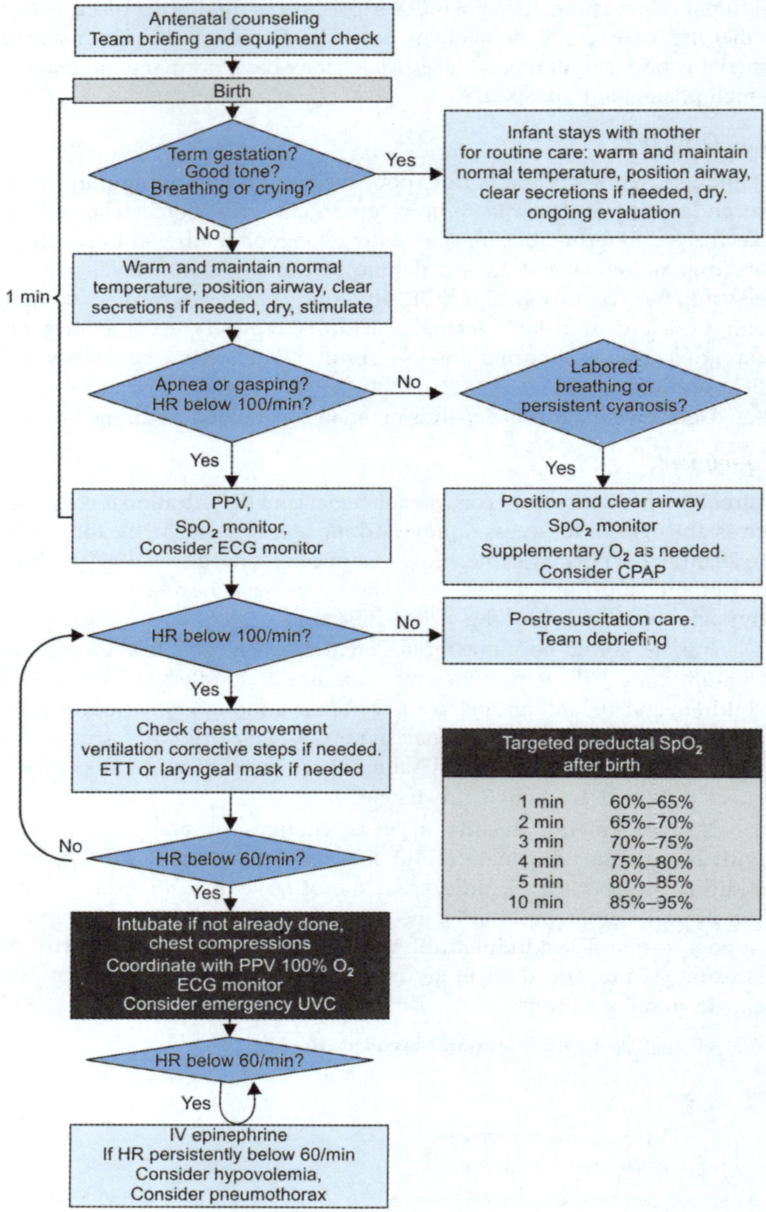

- Most successful indicator of response to resuscitation is increase in heart rate. An electronic cardiac monitor is the preferred method for assessing heart rate.

10. Which of the following genes is implicated in the pathogenesis of juvenile myoclonic epilepsy?

a. FMR-1
b. Fibrillin-1
c. CHYNN-1
d. GABRA-1

Ans. d. GABRA-1

Juvenile Myoclonic Epilepsy

This is the most common form of idiopathic generalized epilepsy in older children and young adults. It begins in adolescence, typically around age 15 years, with a range that essentially spans all of the teenage years. The patient comes to attention because of a generalized tonic-clonic seizure, often upon awakening or because of myoclonic jerks in the morning that involve the entire body; sometimes absence seizures are prominent. The family reports that the patient has occasional myoclonic jerks of the arm and upper trunk that is brought out with fatigue, early stages of sleep, or alcohol ingestion. A few patients in our experience have had only the myoclonic phenomena and rare absence or tonic-clonic seizures that persisted unnoticed for years. The EEG shows characteristic bursts of 4- to 6-Hz irregular polyspike activity. A linkage has been established to several loci, mainly of ion channels and of GABA-related receptors. The genes implicated in JME are GABRA-1, EFHC-1, CACNB-4.

The disorder does not impair intelligence and tends not to be progressive, for which reason it has been called "benign," but a proclivity to infrequent seizures usually continues throughout life. A report by Baykan and colleagues has indicated that, over an average of two decades, the majority of patients have long seizure-free periods and a large reduction in myoclonic seizures by the fourth decade but only one-fifth become virtually seizure free. Valproic acid in particular and some other antiepileptic drugs are highly effective in eliminating the seizures and myoclonus but they should be continued indefinitely as discontinuation of medication is associated with a high rate of relapse. Owing to the potential teratogenicity of valproate, women of childbearing age are often given levitiracetam or lamotrigine, acknowledging that they may not be as effective as the first choice of drug. It has been observed that carbamazepine and phenytoin may exaggerate the seizures.